# Break The Crave System

## ...7 Steps To Effortless Lifelong Weight Loss

Bridgette Hamilton

**FIRST EDITION**

GREEN CAT BOOKS

www.green-cat.co/books

BRIDGETTE HAMILTON

# CONTENTS

# ACKNOWLEDGMENTS

My dearest sis Liz- my inspiration and the loveliest 'smug cow' I know! Also my amazing husband Andy "The Gambler" H-G, whose nit-picking skills helped me finish this book. Also, thank you to Lisa Greener, Sarah Banks and Claire Saxton for helping me bring it into the world. Lastly to Dr Lucy Sargisson for her wonderful help and support.

# INTRODUCTION

I stood on the scales with my eyes closed. I didn't want to look, but I knew that I had to see what the damage was this time. I steeled myself to open my eyes, and I looked down and sighed. My heart sank and I groaned inwardly. I could have cried at that horrible feeling of disappointment...no, let's call it what it was by then...hopelessness. Plain and simple. I had put on more weight than I thought, and I'd only lost it a couple of months before. It had all piled back on. Yet again. And then some. Again.

I clearly remember wondering at that moment, if I could possibly go through that horrible torture of struggle, diet, denial and obsession any more...knowing that it would be followed by almost inevitable weight gain. It made me feel anxious, and I was frustrated to the point of desperation. As I looked back over the weeks before, I tried to find the foods that had caused me to slip up so badly. But I didn't really know what I'd done to deserve this Death By Scales and I began to feel really low. I just didn't have any answers for how to generate weight loss that would last.

I had never been hugely overweight, but over the last couple of years it had crept up by a few pounds here and there, until I was over 4 stone heavier. I had tried lots of low-fat diets but after a few weeks I would lose my mojo and give in to temptation when the smallest of issues happened in my life.

If I wasn't losing weight as fast as I wanted to, that would especially give me a reason to pig out "What's the point? I may as well accept that it's not going to happen and learn to love my fat clothes!" Yeah, great reasoning Bridge...but it didn't last long, and then I'd just be gutted with myself and go on another Punishment Binge. And that would be sugar, of course.

I instinctively knew that lowering fat in my diet didn't actually help me to lose weight. It just felt so...*un- natural* to me. So I started to do a little research and put my own training to better use. I'm trained in nutrition and diet, you would think I had all the answers wouldn't you? It's not as simple as that though. I put my energy and expertise into what really might work for me, going against some of the traditional nutrition advice. What did my body really need to lose the weight in a way that felt natural? Comfortable? Right?

*And then it all came together and it literally hit me. I found the 'secret'. The sweet spot.*

And the weight started to drop off! Naturally. Without any effort or starvation dieting. I couldn't believe my luck! I almost didn't trust it because it felt too good to be true. If I ever went 'off plan' with it for whatever reason, I would find myself craving to go back to my way of eating because it felt so good. That had NEVER happened before! I lost 4 stone in a little under 18 months and I had never felt better. I couldn't deny my energy levels, or indeed what the scales were telling me. I never looked back. That was 7 years ago. I had comfortably lost the weight and more importantly- kept it off.

*It felt like a miracle.*

How did I do it? In a nutshell, I combined the training in nutrition, as well as anatomy and physiology, and a geeky amount of research into the chemistry of the body as it metabolises fuel. I'm also a clinical hypnotherapist so I've learned a few tricks that harness the fabulously powerful motivational systems of the brain. I put it all together in one big gorgeous handbag of tools...and created a perfect recipe for success.

*Your body has a secret. In fact it has lots of them, but there is one very big secret that it holds.*

This secret is the reason over 60% of the adult population are carrying more fat reserves than our body needs. This is despite a weight loss industry worth over £1.8 billion. It's despite the fact that at any moment 30 million of us are on a fat reducing diet. And despite advice about how to eat to lose weight from a record number of sources of information. GPs prescribe free weight loss club memberships to clinically obese patients. The food industry brings out one 'healthy' food product after another. And yet we're heavier than ever. We're more poorly from the food that we eat than any other single reason in this country.

*This secret has been holding you back from shedding your excess fat cells.*

The secret is simple and easy. The dice have been loaded against you from the very start, because unfortunately there is a vested interest in keeping it from you. I'm no conspiracy theorist, but I'm afraid it's because your misery is worth a lot of money. The dice have been loaded against you for over 40 years.

*Take a look around you. We're getting worse. Not better. Something is clearly wrong. Something is simply not working.*

When you first decide to lose weight, you tell yourself that *THIS TIME* you'll stick to the diet. You won't give in. You'll stay motivated and strong. No matter what. Anyone would think you were singlehandedly scaling a mountain rather than shedding a few fat cells. I mean it can't be that difficult, right? After all the latest diet club will tell you that as long as you follow a few golden rules, you'll be slim and successful. Until you slip.

That one small moment when you give in. And then you slowly slide back down to the bottom of the mountain again. Only this time, you actually find yourself dropping down a deep crevasse, where you pile on even more fat reserves than you were carrying before! The mountain has defeated you. Again.

*What if the secret was actually this? There is no mountain to climb. No mega willpower needed. No need to punish, deny or strive in any way...because your body is actually a fat burning machine.*

And I'm going to show you exactly how to return to that very natural state. To arm you with all the information you need to break the secret code that industries with a vested interest have known about your body for a long time.

*To load the dice in your favour.*

This book is going to teach you exactly how to take back control of your eating habits. Read it all the way through, and it will help you understand why you do what you do, and, more importantly, what to do about it. Then you can go back and dip in to the bits that matter to you.

Get to know the **Break The Crave System** as well as you need to, it really won't take long.

*Then lose the pounds. Keep them off. And go and do something more interesting instead!*

Love Bridgette x

www.breakthrough-weightloss.co.uk

## CHAPTER 1 ... THE DARK POWER OF THE CRAVE!

*"Power's not given to you. You have to take it"* Beyoncé Knowles Carter

### Where to Begin?...

Fat is the antidote to *CRAVE,* and processed carbohydrates, sugar and low-fat diets are the trigger.

I know I'm getting a little ahead of myself here with that statement, so let me explain by first of all telling you what *CRAVE* is....and how you know you've got it.

In fact, I think I'm still a little too far ahead of myself, so just bear with me while I backtrack a few years! I need to let you know about my Little Sugar Addiction.

I didn't actually realise I was a sugar addict until fairly recently. I just thought I was a greedy pig that couldn't resist the sugar. I thought I should be able to. After all, my sister could...she could just have *one* chocolate out of a shiny box she had as a pressie then put the rest back in the fridge...Smug Cow. Me? I'm thinking, "Wait till you've left the kitchen sis, those chocs are MINE!" ("You clearly don't want them, do you? Or you'd have eaten the whole lot straight away, in one go, without stopping for breath, wouldn't you?")

Around 15 years ago, my daughter was very poorly in hospital. She was just 6 years old and it was Easter time. Her appetite was gone, and especially so for sugary chocolate. The Easter eggs from caring relatives sat in the fridge, waiting for her to get well. In my defence, I did at least ask:

"Lou, you know how poorly you feel, and you don't want to eat your Easter eggs?"

"No I don't want them Mummy, my tummy hurts!"

"Well, can I eat them for you instead?"

And my little chicken replied, "Yes mummy, of course you can"

And I did. I ate them all up.

And Lou still reminds me of the time I ate her Mars Bar...she was about 8 and only allowed sweets from the shop (of course!), because they weren't kept in the house. (No point!). So we went to the shop and she bought a Mars Bar as a special big treat with her money. Only she was riding her bike, so she couldn't carry it back home:

"Will you carry it for me mummy?"

"Yes darling, of course I can."

By the time we'd got home, you can guess where that Mars Bar was, right? Strangely, nowhere to be found. We had to go and get another one. I felt a bit too sick to eat that next one anyway, much to Lou's relief. Poor kid.

Around that time when my daughter was still quite young, I was cleaning houses as a way to bring in some money as a single parent. I was very good at it because I loved it. I particularly loved knowing that when the working woman of the house walked through the front door, the first thing she would see would be the vacuum stripes in the carpet. I could imagine her relief and pleasure in that. I was so good at my cleaning business that I had a waiting list, and I charged clients by the house, rather than an hourly rate. I was energetic too...luckily! I rode a bike to work and was really quite fit.

I would often clean 3 houses in a day, and travel to them all on my bike. So luckily weight wasn't an issue. I really made the connection in those days with how important it was to move your body to keep your metabolism up. But more than that, I knew how *happy* it made me feel. Cycling around the highways and tracks around Nottingham is still my therapy time today, and I've prioritised it to the point that I'm no longer a fair-weather girl. I'll risk all kinds of tricky weather forecasts to get my morning hour on the bike a few times a week.

As far as those days were concerned, I have stories that could fill a confession booth for a fortnight, and a good proportion of them would be about how my poor clients left chocolates around. Especially at Christmas time...were they mad?? The chocolates would have to be sampled and savoured as I went about my cleaning work. After all, what's a 'couple' of little wrapped choccies? They would have offered them to me if they had been there, I'm sure! The funny thing is, most of my clients *gave* me chocolates whenever they bought me a 'Thank You' present. Those presents hardly ever made it home. They were gobbled up while I worked - and the wrappers were very carefully hidden in the big bin so they didn't think I was a greedy pig.

## My Catalogue of Disgraceful Sugar Stories Could Fill the Pages of This Book...

For example, I remember a time when Lou was very small, around 18 months old, and I was on 6 bars a day. I just couldn't seem to satisfy the craving for sugar for very long. I would then have periods of being 'good' - for a while. I would go on a calorie-reducing diet and I would wear heavy Pretend-Blinkers on my eyes so I just couldn't see that sugar. But all my best efforts would be down the drain if I took the sneakiest peek and noticed the enticing sugary smell, or, heaven forbid - someone actually *offered* me chocolate. That was downright *permission!*

And then it would be as if I'd never abstained and I'd eat the lot... of whatever sugar was in front of me at the time... and it didn't necessarily have to be mine, just fair game. It simply wouldn't stand a chance! And then I would need some more. And then I couldn't stop. I would wake up the next morning feeling awful, with a sugar fog in my brain.

My body heavy and drained. Feeling lethargic, and too stodged to eat breakfast. But I would be full of resolve and feeling strong that I was *not* going to eat the sugar today! Today would be different.

And then something would happen at around tea time. (Or earlier, but around 4 ish seemed to be the golden hour.) I would just cave in completely and eat whatever sugar I could lay my hands on. Sometimes I would find myself going out of my way, of literally putting everything else on hold, until I had eaten some sugar. Including sugar sandwiches. And lemon curd sandwiches. There were never really any sugar products apart from that in my house because they simply wouldn't last. There was just no point. I was either keeping it out of the house for my own protection, or I had trawled my way through whatever was there in one sitting.

Sugar was my enemy, but I still had no real idea of how much it had a hold on me.

I blame my mother really.

(We all do!).

I was a child of the '60 s and all the shops shut at 5 o' clock. Except on Wednesdays when they shut at 1 o' clock. I had a 10p mix on a Friday, and rice pudding on a Sunday. That was my lot. Simply no other sugar around. Unless you count the sugar sandwiches for tea, that is, or the odd cake (my mum wasn't exactly Fanny Craddock though, so no Victoria sponges for us...and funnily enough...I don't particularly feel much for sponge either way). And there was, of course, Carter's pop delivered to the door in various Additive-Neon blues, greens and reds.

And that was it. I was completely sugar deprived apart from that. My whole generation were. As were the ones before us. Because if we wanted to be greedy sugar pigs, it simply wasn't there. So we ate what we were served in our meals instead. And we actually didn't *feel* deprived in the slightest. It was just how it was, and nobody around me knew any different. Sugar addiction simply *did not* exist, because there wasn't enough of the supply!

## It Was The Way It Was ...

Adults would use sweets as a treat, or to console, comfort, cajole, blackmail or commiserate...there was absolutely no harm in it at all, because that would be the end of the story.

We would gobble down our ill-gotten gains or tokens of affection, and then get over any minor subsequent cravings we might have had in the following days and just get on with enjoying our tea. Sweets became treats, a currency the adults around would use to barter with us. They had a kind of *power* in our lives, even a sort of reverence, as the occasions we could enjoy them were so rare.

(It might be difficult to grasp this concept today, as sugar is so readily available now, but I suppose you can compare it to how rare and precious salt used to be. It's a fact that Roman soldiers were actually paid in salt, and it's where the word *salary* originates from. Now of course, it's everywhere, and causing almost as many problems to our health!).

If one of us had sweets on the park, all the kids would crowd round in the hope of them getting divvied out, or they might manage to snatch one for themselves if they were lucky. As we grew older and wiser, the rules would change. If you had sweets, you avoided your friends until you had no more. You would find a quiet secret place to gobble them down all to yourself. Every last bit. And you wouldn't even think twice about it. They were a prize and something to be kept to oneself. The secretiveness was part of the forbidden pleasure...the chance to take something off and huddle it to you, something that was all yours that no one could take away from you or make you share.

**The Rule of the Playground.**

Me and my sister would rarely be given sweeties as a treat, so the Christmas Chocolate Selection Box was something to be speculated on for weeks before....Curly Wurly and a Fudge bar was a definite...but what about a

Caramac? Or one of the big guns like a Marathon or Mars bar? We knew there would be spangles, but you just had to accept that. A bonus would be a packet of chocolaty sweets like Mintolas or Rolos. How long would the box last for me? Not long. About the same amount of time as the chocolate Christmas tree decorations as soon as everyone had left the room. Five minutes. Tops. Well, maybe a day for the selection box. After all I was still only young. The food industry hadn't yet caught on to the golden dream ticket of *CRAVE*. We were spared all of that.

As I read back over this chapter, I realise that if I substituted any number of substances into those stories...alcohol, cocaine, or other harder, meaner drugs... and my out of control, sneaky, all-or-nothing, downright untrustworthy behaviour would be seen as addictive wouldn't it? I'm a therapist and my colleagues and I, we would say that right off the bat, "You're an addict, mate, and I can help you with that," yet it took me *forever* to realise that it was the same for me with sugar.

We're all starting to twig now, aren't we? You can get addicted to sugar. I have never before or since had such out of control urges as I have had with sugar. I was an addict, but all I thought was that I just needed a little more will power. Like everyone else seemed to. If I could just get a little control over myself, I wouldn't *want* sugar any more. If I wasn't so weak, I could *somehow* do it. I could resist and just have the one and put the box back in the frid~ could say, "No thank you I'm full,," I could ta~ Or just leave it and say "Oh that's far too could be a smug cow. *Somehow!*

Now I'm a little better informed and I can see why it's easy to substitute any other highly toxic, incredibly addictive chemical into my addiction story - because sugar is just that: it's an addictive substance. It is just as addictive as other, nastier substances, in fact in some ways even more so. And it's much harder to handle because it is in *everything*.

## How Did This Happen?...

*One day, around 1976, members of the food industry, and the scientists working in their labs, had a wonderful revelation, the marvellous misery of slavery that so many of us would be yoked to- they discovered that they could cleverly design their food with a blend of ingredients and textures that would ultimately create a feeling of CRAVE so strong within us that we simply couldn't resist their food, no matter how hard we tried! This was to be the source of all our body misery, and I might even say heartbreak, for many years to come.*

And then the marketers were rolled in.

They began to spend what would eventually reach *billions* on advertising and research and they started touting these products as "Healthy".

"Happy".

"A Little Treat".

The Next Latest Breakfast Thing".

"The Next Latest Health Food Thing".

"Be Good to Yourself" and

"Live Well" and

 "Eat More" coz its "Healthy" and

"Indulgent "and

"It Makes You Feel *Special*".

"You *Deserve* This One".

"This Will Make You *Sexy*".

 "This One's Got Little Bugs In It That Will Somehow Help Your Gut".

"This Will Make You *Strong*".

"If You Give This One To Your Kids, It Will Instantly Make You A Perfect Mum". Or

 "You Will Automatically Become A Wonderful Wife With That One".  Or

"This Will Make You An *Amazing* Hostess".

"All The Family Will *Gasp* At Your Puddings".

"Just Opening The Wrapper Will Make You A Sex Goddess".

"Give This To Your Girlfriend And She Will Think You Are An *Amazing* Boyfriend".

"You're Too Busy To Cook,, So We Will Generously Concoct This Nutritionally Deficient Slop As A Meal For

You".

"The Photo Will Be Fantastic On The Box, Of Course! "

" If You're Happy You Can *Celebrate* with this".

"If You're Miserable, You Can *Commiserate* With This".

"This Will Make You *Thin*".

"This Is *Just The Once* Coz You're Worth It. *Treat Of All Treats*".

"Once You Pop, You Can't Stop".

---

*Although sugar is a huge problem, it's not just that. There are a few more forces than just sugar at work here. You know you don't have to be a sugar addict to be miserable with your weight! You just have to be out of control with your eating, and the sugar in your food has more to answer for than you might realise.*

---

## The List Of Persuasive Advertising Is Endless. Did They Succeed? Do You Buy Them?

If like so many millions of us, you do... have you ever *REALLY* thought why?

The *CRAVE* revolution began its story in the 70's and the food industry hasn't looked back since. And neither has the weight loss industry. Our collective bodies went into *CRAVE* around about that time, and for most of us it's been the story, and the state we have existed in ever since.

*The Evil Twins Of The Food And Weight Loss Industry Have Tricked Us!*

One told us it was the answer to our food prayers, and our busy lifestyle demands - the other claimed it was the answer to our clearly under-motivated, self-indulgent, weak-willed weight prayers. They promised, "Just do what we tell you and you *won't ever* be fat again!" Now I'm no conspiracy theorist, but there's something you need to know. They were, and still are, lying. Or advertising, you might call it. Plain and simple. In chapter 3 I'm going to explain what has been going on in your body, just so you can understand a little more fully what these companies already know about you.

## In The Rest of This Book...

I'm going to explain why you're miserable that you can't lose weight and keep it off. Why, in fact, you end up gaining even more over time. And you know what? If I know these things about your body, then I can bet every single body-weight of Cadbury's cream eggs that I have ever scoffed that the multi-*billion* pound food and weight loss industries know this about your body too.

And those two industries spend many millions a year on getting into your psychology to tell you that it's *YOU* that's the problem. And you don't get a minutes' training in defence of all that!

*It's Time to Re-Claim Your Body Right Back to Where it Belongs...Under The Control of YOU!*

I'm going to put you right and show you how it is actually the simplest and easiest thing in the world. I will show you step by step, exactly how to do that. There *is* a way. I've called it the **S.P.E.C.I.A.L** system. It is the Break the Crave System and all I'm going to ask is that you commit to taking those steps: Don't worry...they are very easy.

Then over the next few weeks you will begin to feel like you just woke up out of a fog. You will realise one day that you had a feeling, and you didn't really even know it was there - and now you're free of it.

You're free to make your own choices about what to eat. And how much. And when. And you'll not stress about food any more.

You might even find you don't quite know what to think about so much in the mornings at work. Because you won't be going over every regretful mouthful that you picked at last night. Trying to work out how many calories were in it. And how you're going to just succeed today, and what exactly you're going to eat. And how many calories there are in it.

 If you want to know more about me and even more details about how I do all of that...then visit www.breakthrough-weightloss.co.uk.  By all means! I think I'm going to put on a sparkling purple cape and call myself Liberator Gal...to the Rescue!

*In the following five chapters, I will explain why and how we CRAVE and how you can beat it.*

*In the next chapter I'm going to explain how your body goes into CRAVE and in chapter three...how this reflex affects your food choices.*

*In chapter four, you'll get to understand why the food you eat is making you overweight.*

*Then in chapter five I'll show you the seven simple and easy steps to take yourself out of the CRAVE state.*

*How to bring it into your daily life and make it a permanent part is in chapter six.*

*So let's begin by finding out what's been going on behind the scenes ...*

## *Try This Simple Exercise...*

If you're not sure whether you're addicted to sugar, then take a piece of paper and write down the last time you ate or drank it (as in fizzy or sweet fruity drinks, not tea or coffee) This exercise is just for sugar....we'll go into processed carbs later in the book.

Now write down the last few times you've eaten it or had a sugary drink and over what period of time. How many days are there in between the times you had sugar? Is there a regular pattern there?

Once you've got a little picture of the pattern of your sugar intake over the last few days, write your answers to these 10 questions *honestly:*

If you've answered 'yes' to more than 2 or 3 of them (and if you've answered 'yes ' to number 10 alone), then we can safely say that you're a sugar addict. Don't worry...you won't be for much longer!

1. Do you wake up in the morning (more than once or twice out of a week) determined not to eat any sugar but give in and eat it anyway? You might then feel disappointed or ashamed with yourself afterwards (but not necessarily!).

Yes/No

2. Do you decide you're just going to eat 1 chocolate out of the box, or just a couple of biscuits or otherwise limit the amount of sugar, and then eat far more than you intended?

Yes/No

3, Do you buy it for others whilst out shopping and then eat it for yourself instead (*especially* if you secretly knew you were going to eat it for yourself all along)?

Yes/no

4. Do you have All-or-nothing-thinking with sugar? Such as:

i) I've eaten a few chocolates/ biscuits etc already so I may as well eat all the rest, or

ii) I've gone 'off plan' and eaten rubbish, so I may as well carry on for the rest of the day and start again tomorrow, or

iii) I'll just eat everything that's in the house, and then it will be all gone and I can start again tomorrow (There are LOTS of others, but you get the idea!).

Yes/No

5. Do you have a hidden stash of sugar, *NO MATTER* what excuse you give? "I'm hiding it so the kids don't eat too much" is *NOT* the real reason you're hiding it. It's a STASH, and you're concealing sugar from others for different, more personal reasons.

Yes/No

6. Do you think about sugar when you're in the middle of something else, when you didn't want to think about it? And/or do you have out-of-control thoughts about sugar that just won't go away?

Yes/No

7. Do you go out of your way for it?

Yes/No

8. Do you cut calories out of your daily diet, or even cut out meals altogether because you've binged on sugar earlier in the day?     Yes/No

9. Do you eat other people's share, with or without their knowledge?

Yes/No

10. Do you 'sneaky' eat when no one else is around for the sole purpose that you don't want anyone else to see you doing it?

Yes/No

## CHAPTER 2... WELCOME TO THE PLEASUREDOME!

*"God may forgive your sins, but your nervous system won't!" Alfred Korzybski*

## Hardwired for Sugar...

You don't have to be a sugar girl to be in *CRAVE* of course. Not everyone is, but we *are* hardwired to seek out sugar.

It's part of our deep survival programming to feed it to our bodies because it's a superstar rocket fuel. It hits the bloodstream at 1000 miles an hour for an instant starburst of energy.

Sugar is a highly rarefied fuel that will inject a blast of energy into your body so strong that your pancreas won't actually know how much insulin to make in order to deal with it. And will often produce far more than your body actually needs to process it.

---

*We would have trekked miles and miles for sugar in centuries past.*

*We would have risked being stung by outraged bees as we found ourselves a juicy, sticky bee-hive or we stumbled across the fallen Autumn fruit. We got very clever at knowing where these little caches of golden sugar heaven were, and would closely guard the secret, I would imagine.*

*The Rule of the Playground.*

---

And then that was it. Then it would be gone.

And we would go back to our usual sources of fuel and be very healthy on that. We might have had a sugar dip in the next day or so, and maybe even snap at our offspring or mate. We might have a sugar fog and forget what day it was. We might even have experienced a fleeting *CRAVE* for it and wished we could have it again. But that wouldn't last long, because our body would feel very satisfied with its usual sources of fuel, and we would forget all about sticky golden nectar after a short space of time.

Our body chemistry would return to its normal, satisfied state and the rocket fuel would be a sweet and delicious memory.

## Your Nervous System...

This deep programming is still running the show for you.

It is your nervous system and she is *not* to be messed with! She is actually at the heart of nearly every decision you ever make in your life and she doesn't care what sized jeans you want to wear...*her* job is to keep you alive! She will ensure that her messages are your absolute top priority in every single situation. *EVER.* Have I said that emphatically enough?!

Her messages are nerve messages.

And they race through your body at the speed of light. That's the fastest thing in the universe. Nothing faster. Especially not your thinking processes.

Conscious thoughts are a relatively recent addition to our biology and they are *10 times slower* than your nervous system messages.

*You know that thought, when you tell yourself you don't want to eat that piece of cake/chocolate/biscuit/ or those crisps..*

*Or that enormous pile of mashed stodge...*

*Or the kids' leftovers...*

*Or your friend's chips...*

*And you're actually telling yourself "I don't want to eat this!" as it's going in your mouth...*

*And you're thinking "But I'm full, and I don't want this!" and it's going in anyway?*

*That's your nervous system MAKING YOU EAT...YOU don't run the show. SHE does. So you'd better make friends with her. Sharpish.*

This is the programming we are working with, and this is what the food and weight loss industry know about your body. *They have designed their success around it.*

So how do you take control of your nervous system? How do you lift yourself out of *CRAVE* and back into forgetting all about the food that seems so utterly irresistible to you right now? Let's just say that our bodies haven't changed that much in the last couple of thousand years, so what made us feel fulfilled, satisfied and content all that time ago is exactly what makes us feel the same today.

Most of us just don't know this, of course. I've had a geeky fascination with our body chemistry and nervous system, and the way it drives our eating behaviour for a long time. Most people don't make it their business to find out about this kind of thing because they've got lots of better things to do with their time.

I don't blame them, but the trouble is, we trust the 'experts' to tell us how to lose the pounds.

*The 'experts' tend to range from not completely fully informed in their information, to simply deliberately misleading... for whatever reason (usually financial!).*

In the last 50 years, there has been highly dubious 'evidence' from very unreliable science about what is good and bad for our bodies as far as weight loss is concerned. I'm not going to get too geeky about this, but you do need to know just a little about what's going on with you and your nervous system. Then you will be armed with all the information you need to take back control.

And then *you* will be back in control, working with, not against her.

## Your Nervous System and Stress...

She rules your body. Her messages vary in degrees of volume and intensity, depending on what she needs you to know. When you're feeling stressed, it's because your nervous system is having trouble processing all the information you're taking in at any one moment.

That's not to say that we can't cope with *any* stress, in fact we are designed to do just that, but we just can't cope with the *amount* of information and decisions we have to cope with in this modern age.

*Your Body Has Adapted To Thrive On A Certain Amount Of Stress.*

At its finest, stress is stimulating. It helps you to rise to challenges and to enjoy a pleasurable sensation as you achieve your goals. It helps us succeed in our careers and it pushes us to set 'personal bests' in exercise.

*It Helps Us To Excel As Human Beings And Become What We Choose To Be.*

At our best, it takes us out of our comfort zone and into the exhilarating freedom that awaits us on the other side. This is the kind of sensation we feel that is positive and life affirming, it makes us feel strong and unstoppable.

*This feeling happens in your solar plexus. It's a very particular spot just below your ribs where there is a huge bundle of nerves.*

It is the receiver of messages from your nervous system. If you're clever, and you want to continue to do well, you can train your mind and body to re-create these wonderful feelings using NLP, self-hypnosis, and personal development training. On a good day.

## On A Bad Day, However...

there is a message that is sent to exactly the same place, by exactly the same system, only this is a message of discomfort. For some people it can rise in volume to a screaming force of terrible, dreadful alarm. This triggers panic attacks and even Post Traumatic Stress Disorder. It can feel like an unremitting insistent blaring that haunts us with a terrible sense of urgency. And it is absolutely dreadful.

It triggers conditions of the nervous system that are so draining that I am in awe of those who carry on running their lives suffering this background hum of alarm. Most sufferers will hold down jobs and raise families, but the price is terribly high: there is very little joy, and often years of debilitating mental distress. There are many heroes among us who manage to bear these conditions and carry on. They are some of the bravest people I've ever met.

But for most of us, most of the time, we receive a very mild stress message, and we receive this in our solar plexus with the odd 'threat' signal thrown in for good measure.

When for example, we have to stand in front of other humans on a stage and - *talk!* Urrhhh!

## The Amygdala ...

Your Amygdala is the little gland that runs the whole show.

She comes into her finest moment when you're walking past a dark alleyway - you're about to wander down it and for some reason the hairs rise like hackles on the back of your neck and you have an unexplainable fear about it. It just doesn't *feel* right. So you keep walking right on past. Chances are that the deeper part of your mind, your subconscious- has spotted a shadow moving just below your conscious alert senses.

Your subconscious actually runs your Amygdala and all your body's functions for you, so you can get on with running your day. So your Amygdala picked up the message in less than a millisecond and stopped you in your tracks. Saving you from who knows what.

She is also behind that same message you feel when you meet a man and you just don't trust him for some reason. But there's probably a 50/50 chance of us not taking any notice of *that* one, now isn't there?!

---

*This amazing variety of nerve signals is sent by the same part of our brain to our solar plexus, at the same lightning speed. The messages are unbreakable, unshakeable and utterly undeniable.*

*We NEVER ignore our solar plexus, because we're just not designed that way.*

---

In fact the whole messaging system is an unbreakable circuit. Why? Because its job is to keep you alive, out of trouble, with all your basic survival needs met. These basic needs include:

Food.

Fluid.

Shelter.

Protection.

Safety.

Social inclusion.

Connection and approval.

Comfort and nurturing.

Rest and relaxation.

Play (yes, really!)

....And habit.

It doesn't seem like much, but these basic needs are what we run on.

Every single day. Without exception or rule.

These things get met first and last, the more basic they are, the more likely they are to be met first. Basic survival is a very impulsive affair, that's why a nerve signal is so much quicker than the conscious 'human' part of our brain. Because our survival is something that must happen. In the moment. No messing about.

Suppose you had a dinosaur running towards you at 100 miles per hour: you're not stopping to wonder if it's a vegetarian or a meat eater, are you? Your brain says "scram!" and you've scrammed before you've even had time to think. Literally. Have you ever had that experience where you jumped when someone was standing behind you? Even though in that split second you had actually recognised them as friend? That same, lightning speed circuit is in play.

## Survival versus Goal Setting...

This survival system is at odds with the 'goal setting' part of your brain. The part of your brain that has plans. The part of you that makes decisions for the future.

In particular, for this book, it's the part of you that has a Body Goal for yourself.

It is very good at strategy and has the ability to vision another time in your life where you will have achieved your goal.

It's actually a relatively recent addition to your brain function, and is the part of you that mainly deals in a 'thinking' capacity. In its own right, it can be a very powerful function indeed, and will work incredibly well for you.

But in a way, you might call it a 'luxury' when compared to the in-the-present-moment reactions of your survival system. The survival system will cancel out all 'luxury' thinking if it perceives impending threat (in your case, the primal need to feed yourself).

*You need to know that now. Your survival system is 100% dominant, because its job is survival, and it exists in this single moment. There's no 'future' awareness in this circuit. Just instant reaction.*

These two circuits are the ones we are interested in and have everything to do with your weight loss. And gain.

Unfortunately, the clash in priorities of these two circuits means that unless they are somehow synchronised and working harmoniously, they will be as likely to help with your Body Goal as the telly ads in between the soaps.

*Not. In any way at all.*

They simply can't communicate with each other. What this means for you is that setting a goal and sticking to it must take into account the fact there is another, more powerful part of you that is programmed to sabotage your every dream for your Body Goal. There *is* a way to harness this power:

All it takes is a little foresight (or some Insurance Policies, let's call them) and I'll teach you all about these in chapter 5.

---

*This perfectly designed survival system of yours is run by a little gland in your brain.*

*It is a little radar, constantly tuning itself to all the information being picked up from the outside world and the messages from inside your body.*

*It has absolutely no logic, and not one ounce of negotiating will work with it.*

---

We don't have dinosaurs running towards us at 100 miles an hour any more. We don't need to light a fire at the front of the cave to ward off predators. We don't have to worry about warmth, shelter, clothing, or the survival of our children.

Your Amygdala hasn't been informed about these comfortable states of affairs, though. She's still got a job to do, and she is going to *DO IT*. She will find perceived threat and let you know about it in less than a heartbeat, so you react quick enough to stay on your toes.

So ...we have spiders that make us scream our heads off at embarrassing moments in front of strangers. Or we feel bullied by the slightest out-of-turn remark. Or we worry about the bills not being paid on time. The kids not doing so well at school. Gravy down the front of your blouse just before an important meeting. A so-called friend telling others not nice things about you.

Heights.

Flying.

Lifts.

Needles.

Steps.

Masks.

Snakes.

Night.

Day.

Thunder.

Rain.

Sun.

Exams.

Crowds.

Silence.

Noise.

And on and on and on she goes, with ten thousand phobias and limitless reasons for anxiety. And many more besides.

## So Now You Get The Picture...

She's a Force of Nature and *AWESOME* in her power. And yet she is absolutely tiny. Shaped like a walnut and nestling above your brain stem, you might overlook her if her voice wasn't so unbelievably *LOUD!*

Her messages are unrelenting and often confusing to us. One minute you're feeling like you want something, then half an hour later you decide you want completely the opposite thing. And often you have no idea why!

*Summary:*

*Your nervous system, sending signals at the speed of light to your solar plexus, is run by a radar gland called the Amygdala, and this gland absolutely runs the show.*

*It always has and it most probably always will.*

*Most of these messages are sent to alert you to a perceived threat.*

When the Amygdala senses the threat of *starvation*, it's nerve message will drive you to reach for sugar (or processed carbs, they are the same thing to your body).

Let's call this the *REACHING* mechanism.

This little message has undermined your best efforts at weight loss for your whole dieting career.

Welcome to the power of *CRAVE*.

*This exercise will be a real eye opener for you when you look back over it in the weeks to come...*

Being able to take charge of your 'stress message' is a trick we should be teaching in schools these days in my opinion!

It doesn't have to be complicated, and you don't have to sit in the lotus position for hours (unless you want to!). This deceptively simple little trick is one of the most powerful tools there are for coping with the stress messages from your nervous system and helping you re-gain a bit of balance.

It will also help you in the long-term, as far as weight loss is concerned, as it will give you a head start in listening to your body's messages without necessarily having to act on them straight away.

---

Find a quiet place to do this exercise, it will only take 10 minutes.

Be gentle with yourself. Take a 'soft' approach to your thoughts, don't judge them, just be aware of them...

CLOSE YOUR EYES:

(PRACTICE WITH MILD FEELINGS AT FIRST WHILE YOU GET USED TO DOING THIS)

1.  Have a think about the last time you felt stressed. can you *FEEL* where it is in your body?
2.  What was your thinking that went along with it?
3.  Did that thinking make you feel *better* or *worse?*
4.  Write down your thinking

**NOW GO BACK TO THAT STRESS MESSAGE AGAIN. REALLY *FEEL* IT FOR A MOMENT**

Don't try and do anything to avoid it or change it. Just notice it. Keep with it until you start to notice it change in intensity.

1. What is your thinking with it now?
2. Does it make you feel better or worse?
3. Write it down.

Try it with another stress feeling you've had recently and see how this exercise can work for it.

Can you feel the difference when you really sit on your own shoulder and *notice* that stress message?

This is a very simple mindfulness practice. If you only do 10 minutes a day, over the course of a few weeks you'll begin to notice the benefit in managing your stress levels.

In fact I can confidently say you will be amazed at how much stress you're able to get on top of (*and* how much stressful thinking you actually have in a day!).

## CHAPTER 3... HOW THE REACHING MECHANISM WORKS

*"Between stimulus and response there is a space. In that space is our power to choose our response. In our response lies our growth and our freedom."* Viktor E. Frankl

## How To Find The Crave Message...

The *CRAVE* message is just as powerful as the threat feeling. But your solar plexus deals with *this* one in a different kind of a way. The message gets scrambled a little, so you don't hear it properly. In fact, you *really* don't hear it *at all*. Well, you don't *register* that you do. It's far too clever for that.

*This Is An Altogether Different Kind Of Sensation.*

This is your survival remember, so your Amygdala cleverly *hides* the sensation and it almost goes under your radar. It can't take the risk of you starving accidentally. You might find that you can put off *REACHING* for food for a while and have an element of conscious control over it. But that can never be for long. Your survival is far too important to be left to *you!*

So the message is delivered in a way so that you think it's something else. You think it's your thoughts. You think it's *you*. You don't register this message because it is *TINY*. And all the more deadly serious for it. It's the cleverest design there is in your body because it completely fools you into thinking it's something else. It fools you into thinking that you're running things! That you *have a say* in things!

And we know how *that* one works out don't we??

Remember the cream cake/chocolate/biscuit/crisps/chips coming towards your mouth?

And you telling yourself you don't want it?

*WHY* don't you put it down?

*WHY* don't you listen to *you*?

*WHY* are you completely unable to stop that *REACHING* mechanism in mid-reach, and change your mind about that food?

After all, you're full. You don't even like the taste of Haribos. Or that cheap brand of crisps that you make out you would never eat.

*WHY* don't you just say,

"No thanks, I'm ok for now, I'm full."?

*WHY* don't you just lose that weight, be done with it, and move on to something more interesting instead?

The reason you don't do this is that you *can't*. This tiny little message goes under your radar, so that you *don't* spot it. It's really so you don't have to think about it. In fact, you barely notice that you've eaten that 6 pack of crisps, or the whole family sized bar.

Or the kid's leftovers. Until you look down and see empty plates, packets and shelves, and then you wonder how that ever happened.

Sometimes you didn't even realise you were eating so much until it had all gone because you'd been absentmindedly grazing on whatever was in front of you. This often happens when you're slightly bored or distracted, in front of the telly or when you're occupied in another task. And this is the most lethal kind of *REACHING* there is because you can eat a whole day's worth of calories in one sitting without stopping for breath.

The *REACHING* mechanism is just another habit that your body has that is designed to serve you, so that you can get on with the business of the day. Then you don't have to consciously think about selecting the right fuel for your body at the right moment. This is left to your subconscious mind and the Amygdala under its influence.

*We literally don't know what happens sometimes. You look at the giant sized empty crisp packet. Or look down at your plate and see that ALL the pudding has gone, when you only intended to have a couple of mouthfuls.*

*Then you tell yourself,*

*"I have no self-control! I'm just like my mother and I deserve to be fat!"*

*Or you realise that you cleared all the kids' leftovers before they got to the bin, when you'd SWORN to yourself that you wouldn't do that tonight!*

*"Well I may as well pig out all evening now I've blown the diet on foraging the leftovers!"*

*See? Where is the control? In your thoughts? Clearly not!*

## *Are You Just GREEDY?...*

So let's clear something up right now. No. You are *NOT* greedy. You are *NOT* weak-willed.

You are *NOT* a failure at everything. You are *NOT* stupid.

You aren't even de-motivated or disheartened.

You are *NOT* an emotional eater.

You are *NOT* a comfort eater either.

You are *NOT* a lazy eater and you probably don't have a particularly slow metabolism (if you actually do have a physical issue...please excuse my poetic license...however you are *STILL* not a done deal!).

You *DON'T* inherit these genes from your granny.

You *DON'T* eat to fill a void in your life.

You are *NOT* just someone who's always been fat.

**YOU ARE NOT TO BLAME AND YOU HAVE NOT FAILED!!**

You *DIDN'T* eat pizza because of self-sabotage issues and you are *NOT* beyond help.

You are *NEVER* beyond help.

You are simply not in control. That is all. Any of the factors and influences above may well have a part to play in your psychology. I'm not doubting that for one moment, and I'm not in *any* way belittling your life experience.

> *What I'm saying is that you REACH because you have a little tickle in your solar plexus that tells you to. But you don't notice that tickle.*
>
> *You concentrate on the thinking part of you so that sensation goes under the radar. Remember how fast that nerve signal is? Yep that's right: the speed of light. Before you've even had a chance to say, "noooooo!!!" It's gone.*
>
> *Gulp. Like one of those lizards with the amazingly fast unravelling tongue.*

That's you, that is. And me. It's every single one of us under the influence of *CRAVE* - and her evil twin sister - *ADDICTION.*

But we are going to fight this. We're going to use every single thing you know about yourself and your little triggers to help you understand where that little tickle came from so that you can let go of it and feel *quiet* in your solar plexus, because when you're quiet, you're done. Plain and simple.

There *is* a way for you, and you *can* take back control! The whole of the rest of this book will be dedicated to that one little moment in your day, when you realise you *don't* want that pudding etc. and you can just say,

"I'm alright for now, thanks."

That's all there is and all there ever is. Nothing else is needed. Just a glorious new way of eating. No latest and greatest diet. In fact, no more diet *ever!* No strategies, methods, or weekly meetings and discussions of your so-called weaknesses.

No public weigh-ins.

No daily-diet-plans that count every single calorie in every single ingredient.

No latest and greatest healthy meal alternative.

No fat-reducing supplements.

No pills.

Or shakes.

Or drinks.

Or bars.

Or sins.

No will-power.

No determination, driven by support from every weary person around you who has ever heard your:

"This time I'm REALLY determined, like never ever before, to succeed and not fail!"

They've heard that story countless times before.

*The Power of The Mundane...*

> *It's not going to be a very dramatic picture is it? Well, that's because it has to be that way.*
>
> *You know why? Drama doesn't work. It's not sustainable and you can't keep it up.*
>
> *It has to be simple. Every-day. Mundane. Habit. Under the radar routine.*
>
> *That way, you won't have to think about it. In the amount of time it takes your brain to re-wire itself, you'll forget that you ever had a problem with your weight.*
>
> *Then your body will be in EASYBURN.*

*Your Brain Takes Just 3 Weeks To Make Lasting Changes To Your Appetite And Meal Choices.*

Can you believe it's that quick? I know. It just can't be right can it? I mean it just can't be that easy! You've spent your dieting life *STRIVING* to lose the weight and keep it off. It's meant to be difficult, right? Because that's what everybody says! If it doesn't *FEEL* like denial, then you won't lose the weight.

You're not supposed to *really* enjoy the food you eat when you're reducing your fat cells, everybody knows that's just a bit of spin from the weight loss industry to make you feel a teeny weeny bit better about the awful gnawing hunger you're enduring.

However, striving hasn't exactly worked has it? In fact, it seems to have made things a whole lot worse somehow, and now your body is more confused than ever.

She's more reluctant than ever to give up her hard-won fat cells to your latest diet whim. She's had enough of this weight game. This rollercoaster ride of emotions and body chemistry fluctuations. She wants out!

Instead of all that hardship, you're going to start to trust your body and the signals she sends you again. You used to once, you know. You ate what your body truly needed. And then you stopped when you were full. Little ones do that, don't they? And we look at them in wistful envy.

These signals will become your brand new very old indicators. Your *real* diet advice.

If it feels good. I mean *truly* down to your boots good. If it feels so deeply satisfying that you feel like sighing in deep pleasure with the food you're giving to her. You will begin to really *tune in* to your body's messages, then you will be able to identify the actual message of *CRAVE.*

## Let's Get Started...

There's no time like the present, so let's start right now. Do the exercise at the end of this chapter, and you'll be ready to go!

It takes your stomach just 3 weeks to shrink back down to its normal size. And that is a real game changer! Then you simply *can't* each so much. Your appetite will diminish to the point where you will be looking for that hunger, and it simply won't be there, and then you'll wonder where it went, and why?

Your body will begin to feel a satisfaction that it hasn't felt in so long. When you begin to feel that feeling, you will remember that you used to feel it. A very long time ago, and you forgot that you did, and now you can realise that your body has been craving something for all these years without you really being aware of it. But now you are!

*Oh Yes...Now You're Becoming Armed And Dangerous!*

So let yourself off the hook, and let's get on with enjoying the process of taking back control. Of looking forward to your food and your meals without any sense of guilt or sinking disappointment.

Of enjoying every mouthful of your meals, and *never* seeing food as the enemy again.

Of peace. Plain and simple. Of feeling so full, so much of the time, that you start to wonder if you're ever going to feel hungry again!

How nice. It's my reality, and the reality for thousands of happy clients who have been through the Breakthrough WeightLoss System. They forget they ever had a problem.

SUMMARY:

*The CRAVE is that little tickle in your solar plexus that creates the irresistible REACHING mechanism.*

*It's too fast and too powerful for you to resist. It can't and won't respond to your thoughts. Noticing it and quantifying it is the beginning of the battle.*

*Understanding how you got it, and how to take out the 7 Step Break the Crave System against it will ensure that you never again feel out of control for very long.*

*We're now going to ensure that you quickly and easily return to a way of eating that satisfies and delights you.*

Please do check out the website if you're looking for more resources...there's loads there...www.breakthrough-weightloss.co.uk

*For this exercise, we're going to work on the fact that your brain doesn't know any difference between real and imagined...*

**If you imagine something, then your brain acts as if it's actually there.**

Find a quiet moment and close your eyes. Imagine that you have your favourite sugary or processed food in front of you. Notice what it smells like. Anticipate the texture of it as you imagine putting it towards your mouth. Imagine exactly what it's going to taste like.

Think about what temperature it will be as you put it towards your mouth.

---

**Ok. Now.**

- **Notice where you feel that urge to eat that food. Can you feel it in your solar plexus? Can you feel that little tickle?**

Some people tell me it feels like a little pulling or an emptiness.

- **Give it a number now so you can really identify it for what it is - 1 being barely there, and 10 being almost overwhelming - where are you on the scale?**

Can you feel that message from your body now? Can you hear her whisper to you?

---

**THAT, my dearest reader, is your CRAVE...**

- **Just take a moment to sit on it. Just like you did in the exercise in the previous chapter. What thoughts do you have around it?**
- **Write them down. Go back to that feeling again.**
- **Now imagine you're eating your favourite cheese, or chicken skin...or whatever your favourite fatty food is.**
- **Again; anticipate what it will taste like as it comes towards your mouth, and how the texture will feel too.**

Can you notice that feeling in your solar plexus this time? Does it feel more satisfied? Content? Is there a more 'full-filled' feeling with it?

When you really notice what this message from your nervous system feels like...what you would really *prefer* to eat?

## CHAPTER 4... TAKE BACK CONTROL!

*"Knowledge is power" Sir Francis Bacon*

### So How Do We Get Into CRAVE?...

And, more importantly for your weight loss....how can we *get out* of it?

There are 3 processes in your body that will put it instantly into the *CRAVE* state:

1. Sugar addiction

2. Eating processed food

3. Being on a diet

### 1. Sugar Addiction...

**Let's take number 1 first as it is one of the most powerful and pervasive problems we have with our food supply today. By far. This is from my experience working with weight loss clients for over a decade now.**

Sugar addiction is literally a perfect storm of influences on your body chemistry. You have the deep biological programming to find and eat sugar that we talked about in chapter 2. Which is so strong that it's enough to give us addictive urges on its own. When you eat or drink simple or refined sugars (including fruit juices), your blood sugars spike and then dip to very low levels.

*So You CRAVE More Each Day To Ensure Those Levels*

*Stay Topped Up.*

Usually at the same time of day (mid-afternoon ring any bells for you?).

You most likely won't be eating properly too, to make up for the sugar...at the very least, you'll be dieting during the day to compensate. Eating as 'healthily' and low calorie as possible to balance the books with the calories you've taken in from sugar. It can drive and ultimately control that *CRAVE* cycle from the minute you wake up till when you got to bed at night. And be such a deep part of your life that you don't even realise it.

*This Is Where We Get All These Ideas That We Eat Sugar For Other Reasons Besides Addiction.*

That way...we can be an emotional eater...*REACHING* for it when we're emotional.

Or a celebratory eater.

Or a happy eater.

Or a sad eater.

Or a comfort eater.

Or an evening picker.

Or a rebellious eater (oh, yes! We are *such* a little rebel with ourselves, aren't we??) And exactly *who* am I rebelling against I ask myself? Well me, obviously, because, let's face it at my age nobody *cares* whether I ate all the cake or not.

We are sugar sharers with our friends when we go out to eat a meal and it comes time for dessert.

Or for coffee and cake.

Or staying in with a movie together.

We are sugar accepters when nice puddings are made for us.

Or when we're given sugar as a present or a treat from a well-meaning loved one or friend (then we're *obliged* to eat the sugar aren't we? I mean, it would be rude *not* to!).

The trouble is...we can also be sugar hoarders, stealers and crammers.

We can go *miles* out of our way for sugar, even in the middle of the night. We can eat nothing but sugar all the entire day, but *nothing*, so that we don't end up with too many calories inside us.

We can eat till we feel sick, then wait half an hour till the feeling has subsided, then eat all the rest, and then feel sick all over again.

We can eat so much sugar that our taste buds have given up, and we don't even notice the true sweetness of it any more.

We can go through the house like a locust eating every single last bit of sugar that there is to be found (and that includes the children's lunchboxes, neatly packed and ready for the next day...now minus the little chocolate bar treat).

What reason do we put on *that* uncontrollable and guilt-ridden behaviour?

The fact is...all of these beliefs are just one simple thing.

*PERMISSION.* The permission we give ourselves, the excuse, the reason, the just-today-but-it-won't-happen-tomorrow reason that it happened. It's *permissive thinking.* And it is the most important reason that we don't twig onto ourselves sooner that we're an addict. That we are addicted to the most common, and by a mile, the most easily available addictive substance on the planet.

If you recognise yourself in any, or all, of these (I've heard even more wildly serious stories of uncontrollable sugar urges from clients over the years, believe me!) and you take nothing else from this book...*Give yourself a break, and accept that you're an addict...*all the rest will fall into place and you will find peace with yourself. I promise you that!

---

*There is a Kick The Sugar download that's helped thousands of happy sugar addicts who never go near the stuff these days, and have  successfully turned themselves off it.*

*It's on here-  https://breakthrough-weightloss.co.uk/product/kick-the-sugar/*

*If you know it's for you, then please don't waste a single second more by punishing yourself!*

---

## 2. Processed Food...

**Now...Put that sugar into PROCESSED FOOD? And you're *really* in trouble! Even if you're *not* a sugar addict!**

This is food that's designed in a lab. You need to know that. The person that concocted your Be Healthy, Be Good To Yourself, No fat-Low Fat, Indulgent, Simply Special, Luxury Edition Fast Dinner, Pudding, Breakfast, Snack and Sneaky Treat, wore a white lab coat...*not* a frilly apron all covered in flour.

You might see a picture of a sweet white haired old lady on the front of the pack. But I've some news for you. It's not a photo of the cook of that product. It's a very clever visual aid they use routinely to fool you into thinking this is home cooked food. So is the picture of the happy healthy children. The reclining indulgent gorgeous woman. The happy snappy teens. The party loving friends. The healthy wealthy family round the table.

I know you know all that. But you only know it intellectually. You don't *know* it. You don't realise that image is far cleverer than the bit-of-you-that-knows. This image gets into your very psyche. Completely bypassing the bit-of-you-that-knows...to go straight for your emotion centre, and guess what? It sits *right next* to your Amygdala in your brain!

And what does that mean? It doesn't think. It reacts, at lightning speed. Below your conscious attention.

So you grab that indulgent-yet-healthy looking yoghurt off the shelf because you've read the wording that say it's low-fat:

"Good for you"

"Healthy bio"

"Full of natural ingredients"

"Real fruit ingredients"

"It will add to your 5 a day" and you can "BuyOneGetOneFree" this week only.

What it *doesn't* tell you, is that it has *at least* 10 grams of sugar added to every single pot. That it will spike your blood sugar in half an hour and actually make you *hungrier* than you were before.

They tell you that the bread is brown, so it better be better for you. What you don't read, is that the milling process that made the grains into flour ensure that the flour bears *no resemblance* to the grains and contains minimal nutrition value. Most brown bread is simply dyed brown in the manufacturing process!

Our ancestors weren't over-weight at all. They were very healthy and weren't bothered by food-related illnesses such as type 2 diabetes in anything like the numbers we do today!

They were quite probably fitter than most of the younger generation who regularly consume the processed food on offer today.

*The bread up to the 70's was a very different affair from what we eat today.*

*When the food industry discovered the processes that allowed mass production, they changed the milling process of grain so that bread is hardly recognisable to the heavy, dense and much more complex kind of loaf your granny would have eaten*

*(And don't forget that she would have put lard or butter on that...or dripping!)*

This is the behind-the-scenes stuff that they think you don't need to know about. But you do. You really do. There are many processes involved in the design of a new product. I won't bore you with them. But there is one more process that we need to talk about in the interests of weight loss:

The bliss point.

**"The Bliss Point is an engineered combination of sugar, fat and salt that will produce an addictive response in the brain, so that you will seek out that food and eat it till you can't eat any more" Professor Tim Noakes.**

The bliss point is the secret weapon the food industry aim at you with the precision, effectiveness, and insidiousness of a laser-guided missile.

You have no defence from it. None whatsoever. Because it goes straight for the jugular. It creates an unbelievably powerful *CRAVE* .

It goes straight to the very heart of your appetite centres and triggers in the brain that control your behaviour.

Let me just re-iterate that for you- *It controls your behaviour.* You do not stand a chance! You don't have a hope of controlling that. It's not just the rubbish cheap ready meals we're talking about here. It's *everything.* Gregg's sausage rolls have sugar in their pastry. Did you know that? Did you know that they put sugar in peanut butter? Why do you think they put sugar in pizza? Why do you think there are so few foods that *don't* contain sugar?

> *Not only does the sugar in everything appeal to every single sugar addict out there, but the combination of sugar, fat and salt is the design.*
>
> *The whole design.*
>
> *The whole addictive concoction that triggers your brain to release dopamine. And we all love a bit of dopamine because it creates such a great feeling within us...it's literally artificial bliss!*

## That's Nearly The Whole Story, But Not Quite...

The rest of it is the *texture.* And they play with that too.

You know why?

*So You Don't Think That You've Eaten.*

If you don't chew your food a certain amount of times...in other words, if it melts in your mouth...or barely takes any chewing at all, then your brain doesn't actually register that you've eaten.

So you eat and eat and eat.

In fact you eat even when you're telling yourself that you've just eaten.

"How can I possibly be hungry?" you ask yourself, "I've just eaten!"

But your brain won't have picked that signal up yet. It's still waiting to send out the message that you're full. And you will eat an entire pack of Pringles in one go, it will barely touch the sides.

"Once you pop, you can't stop" You've just eaten a 1000 calories. And you're still hungry.

Processed food doesn't sit in your digestive system for very long either...not nearly long enough to keep you feeling satisfied. It literally *drops* through your digestive system, pulling the fat and carbohydrate ingredients with it.

You'll store the fat, and you'll store the residual carbs as fat too. And then you'll be starving all over again. You could be in *CRAVE* from morning till night.

Thinking you're just a greedy pig.

So then you decide it's *diet time* ...and your fate is sealed!

## 3. Starving Your Body...

**Being on a diet is the single worst thing you can do to successfully lose weight. Ever. Period. Don't believe me? Take a look around. *Diets are not working.* Clearly. Unfortunately the diet industry is well aware of this.**

And uses your own nervous system against you. The result can be that you're on a diet almost all of your adult life and end up fatter than when you started all those long years ago. By an absolute mile.

In fact, now you look back on it, you probably realise you weren't really all that fat to start with, but there was so much pressure to be thin! So, as so many of us do, you thought you'd better starve yourself a little so that your weight dropped.

But then for some reason, it all went back on again at some point over the years. Maybe after the first time you lost weight, you might have successfully kept the weight off for quite a while. But then you gained a little, maybe after the kids, or getting content in a relationship. Or you took on a busy job with no time to cook properly.

So then you decide to do what you did those years ago and go on a low-fat-calorie-restricted-diet again.

Only this time it's a bit harder, and it doesn't work quite so well. In fact it's torture, but you stick to it.

*All That Self Denial And Gnawing Hunger.*

But then something goes wrong with it. Maybe you keep a lid on your impulses for a while. But all it takes is one good holiday. Relationship break-up. Christmas. Easter egg hunt. Commiserating blow-out on the day the budgie died. And you're back to square one.

Only *this* time, you've put on even more besides. You're defeated and depressed, so you tell yourself you're happy being fat. Anyway, you're too old for diets.

I'm not saying this is all of us. But it is a lot of us. Too many. Too many stories of misery, deprivation and downright obsession. We live in one of the richest countries in the world. How come we're all starving ourselves?

You probably guessed that this is your Amygdala at work. She senses when you're starving, you see. You might keep a lid on her betrayal of your best efforts for a while. But eventually she *will* make you reach for the fuel she senses you've starved yourself of, and then some. And it will always be the quickest source of fuel for your body!...What's that I hear you ask? Sugar, of course! And processed food. It's never the broccoli is it?

*SUMMARY:*

*Your body chemistry will automatically put you into a state of CRAVE through 3 different routes:*

*Sugar, processed food and the sense that you're starving yourself.*

*All these influences trip your Amygdala into perceiving that you haven't taken in enough fuel.*

*That you're starving.*

*You might be starting to ask if there is ANY light at the end of the tunnel here!*

*Well, yes. Oh yes there is! Praise the fat and pass me my breakfast!*

**KEEP A FOOD DIARY FOR 1 WEEK SO YOU CAN SEE HOW YOUR EATING HABITS AFFECT YOUR DAY-TO-DAY CHOICES...**

You might see that out-of-control- urge to eat sugar happened because you binged out at the same time to day before? Or maybe you ate a lot of processed food one day, and you felt un-fillable the next? (Perhaps even the same day?) Were there days that you didn't eat breakfast...and then you couldn't stop eating at night?

You will notice that your emotions on a particular day will have a part to play, but your eating habits actually have a lot more bearing on your food choices than you realised. Start to pick out patterns with your eating that relate to what you ate, or omitted to eat. Either on the same day or the day before at the earliest.

Keep a diary for as long as you like, but I'd recommend at least a week. Use it throughout the rest of this book as you go through the chapters and uncover more about your own unique eating habits! You'll see that your emotions aren't a *consistent* influence on your eating habits, but your food is!

|  | **Monday** | **Tuesday** | **Wednesday** |
|---|---|---|---|
| **Breakfast** | | | |
| **Lunch** | | | |
| **Dinner** | | | |
| **Snacks** | | | |
| **How did I feel today?** | | | |

**Thursday**          **Friday**          **Saturday**          **Sunday**

## CHAPTER 5... THE BREAK THE CRAVE SYSTEM

*"You always had the power my dear, you just had to learn to use it for yourself!"* Glinda, The Wizard of Oz

This is the 7 step process that will take your body out of *CRAVE*, simply and easily, and will turn it into a fat burning *machine.* If you follow these 7 steps, I guarantee that you will never look back. That you will feel more satisfied, content, and happier in your body than you may have been for years.

Remember what we said in chapter 4- nothing else is required of you! This is enough, and all you will ever need. So you can forget about your weight, and get on with the really important things in your life...like living it to the full! So what are we waiting for?

Use this Break The Crave System for 6 weeks and you will notice a huge difference in your body in just that short space of time!

To make it easier to remember the 7 steps and how to progress through them, I'm calling them **S.P.E.C.I.A.L**...you'll see why as you read on!

## STEP 1...

**Sugar.**

Get it out your life. From today. Reading the labels on your food and getting savvy about where it is. Supermarkets often introduce the smell of sugar through the air conditioning, so you buy it without even realising because that's what you were subtly influenced to do (Smell is a very strong subconscious trigger for us). If you're a sugar addict, now is the time to own it and realise it's not your little treat or your little friend. It's poison in a pretty wrapper.

If you need help with getting over the sugar withdrawal, I'm here for you. As I said, I have an amazing Kick The Sugar download that will *turn* you off the sugar after a week or less of listening. It's very powerful, and combined with the 7 steps will give you complete control over your sugar addiction.

*Here's a link for you to the download:*

https://breakthrough-weightloss.co.uk/product/kick-the-sugar/

## STEP 2...

**Processed food.**

Now you're aware of what food manufacturers do to your food and your body, I'm sure you'll be very happy to at least attempt to boil an egg. Really, you don't have to be an amazing cook to make yourself unprocessed meals. See the list at the end of this chapter with the foods to avoid that interrupt your body's fat natural burning system. This is the perfect place to start.

## STEP 3...

**Embrace the fat**....Every last bit of it!

Butter. Cheese, Chicken skin. Bacon fat. Olive oil. Coconut oil. Avocado. did I say cheese? That needs saying again! *YES! CHEESE!* Nuts. Seeds. Beef dripping. Lamb fat. Nut butters. Nut cheeses (the vegan's best friend!) Oat cream. Pork rind.

There are dozens of websites and Facebook pages dedicated to this way of eating, so investigate it for yourself if you need to, and find out everything you can about 'low carb high fat' as a way of eating. Visit "My Diet-Less Life" and come and join my group of Happy Eaters there. A really good website for information from health specialists is www.dietdoctor.com.

If you're looking for other information, this way of eating is also known as the Keto/ Ketogenic diet, or Ancestral Eating (for a very good reason!) if you want to search on the internet. In fact there are literally thousands of sites and pages dedicated to this way of life now. People become very enthusiastic once they discover it for themselves, as it feels like the answer to every single weight loss prayer they have, so a lot is spoken about it, and there are countless forums you can join for free to find out everything you need to know.

*The Simple Reason This Way Of Eating Works Is That Your Body Burns Fats By Default.*

As I said previously carbohydrate, especially *processed* carbohydrate, interrupts this super elegant, efficient system. Even savoury carbs such as crisps are actually converted into sugars for fuel by your body. *All* the processed food (apart from processed meats and cheeses) comes under the same heading of carbohydrates. They *all* end up being the same fuel for your body.

Your body will *only* burn 2 types of fuel...fat or carbohydrates. There is nothing else. She prefers fat and always has done, (which is why you store fat cells for future use...you don't store carbohydrates do you?). I'm not going to go into the chemistry too much here, though.

In a nutshell, your body is designed to burn fat happily all day as a source of fuel, and it always has done. But if you put too many processed carbohydrates in it, then your body will deal with those first as it senses that they are an inefficient fuel source, and it will store the fat till it's finished using the carbohydrates.

> *If you constantly eat carbohydrates, (either savoury or sweet), you will constantly store fat.*
>
> *Take the carbs out of your diet, it will 'system restore' back to its' own innate ability to be a Lean Mean Fat Burning Machine within the space of a couple of days.*
>
> *It will jump into EASYBURN.*
>
> *Oh, and you will feel more satisfied than you could possibly imagine as you are naturally drawn to fat for comfort and a deep sense of nourishment.*

You may think it's the carbs that comfort you, but actually all they do is just mollify the *CRAVE*. It's *fat* that satisfies. Every single time.

*The simple truth is that FAT STORAGE is bad, and it doesn't happen if we are in EASYBURN. Which is a natural fat burning process, (also known as ketosis). Your body employs this process to burn fat for fuel. If we use fat as a main source of fuel, and don't interrupt the fuel burning process with carbohydrates...we simply don't store the fat... how cool is that?*

That's how clever our bodies are. How efficient they are as a Fuel Burning Machine. Your body will literally eliminate any fat that it doesn't use for fuel if you are in *EASYBURN* mode. It doesn't hang on to it, and it will burn off all your lovely stored fat cells in the process too! Your body was designed to use fat and was never designed to use simple or processed carbohydrates as a main source of fuel...it simply can't cope with them well at all.

So now we are going to put your body into *EASYBURN*. And this is how.

## STEP 4...

### Complex carbohydrate veg.

Embrace all the gorgeous green salad, green leafy veg, low gi (glycaemic index) fruits such as strawberries, blueberries and the like. (Sugary fruit will stall your weight loss for sure, and if you're a sugar girl...well, you'll just lurrve the sugary taste of the fructose won't you? So don't be tempted down that route!)

Investigate what these foods are and get creative with them. There is an amazing variety of food awaiting your exploration! I've put a list of some of the common ones to enjoy towards the end of this chapter. I was chatting to a client on the phone the other day...she said she had been telling her hairdresser all about how she lost her weight, and how she fired the processed carbs out of her diet. Her hairdresser asked her.

"What do you eat then"

Her reply is priceless -

"*Everything else,* just everything else!"

## STEP 5...

**Insurance Policies!**

It's vital to take this one out word for word. Get a piece of paper, write down the policy below, sign it and commit to it! An insurance policy is by nature something you do to *avoid* problems later. This Insurance Policy is the single most important thing you do to make very small changes in your lifestyle that will guarantee success and add up to huge changes later on. Yes...I *guarantee* you will succeed if you use this very simple commitment!

---

*I promise...*

*"To think about my tummy and to eat when my body needs it.*

*To have food available and never starve myself.*

*I especially commit to eat a filling breakfast every single morning"*

---

*NO* excuses! If you were feeding a child, there wouldn't be a higher priority in your universe, right?

There's a very old saying, "Breakfast like a Queen, lunch like a lady and dinner like a pauper". This is the biggest Insurance Policy you have against that evening grazing. feeding your body when she actually *needs* that fuel. This will automatically switch on your brain's satisfaction hormone, leptin.

And you'll feel wonderfully full.

Get used to eating breakfast if you don't at the moment. And a really good one too! Warm if possible, with lots of lovely fat! (think double cream in porridge, or bacon and eggs with stir fried greens in butter. I love cheesy buttery scrambled eggs with half an avocado most mornings.)

## STEP 6...

**Allow mistakes** ...and treat this next few weeks as an *EXPERIMENT.*

This will help you get out of the diet/denial mindset. That way you can make your mistakes, learn from them, and begin to get to know yourself and your body so much more deeply.

The food diary is such a good idea. Keep it for as long as you need to and be really honest in it...you'll learn lots about your food habits. This in turn will teach you what particular Insurance Policies you need to take out for yourself.

> *If you give yourself permission to make a mistake without it being the end of the world, then if you ever do accidentally eat processed food, and later find yourself grazing for no reason in the cupboards...This time you'll know why...You'll feel the tickle of the CRAVE and you'll understand. Sit tight or get help.*
>
> *There's a great tapping technique for cravings on the website, and I'd love to let you have the technique as a freebie! Llearn all about it today...it's a lifesaver for stopping sugar cravings!* www.breakthrough-weightloss.co.uk/tft-for-sugar-cravings

*Part Of This Experimental Period Could Be To Weigh Yourself Less Often.*

I know this could be a hard one for you. But I've seen many a client who weighs herself every single day and then sometimes finds herself stuck at that number she sees on the scale. It's almost like your body holds herself to that number. Another good reason is because you won't lose weight at the traditional 2-lbs-a-week slimming-club-way...

It may take a couple of weeks for the scales to start showing the difference in your body and you wouldn't want it to de-motivate you early on. Don't take that chance! Give yourself a month off if you possibly can.

You could see it as a gift to your future self at the end of the month. What a pleasant surprise that will be for you when you see a significant drop on the scales!

Make Insurance Policy number 2:

> *I promise....*
>
> *"To treat this as an experiment and to take myself out the denial/diet mindset"*

# STEP 7...

## Listen to your body's messages!

Begin a two-way conversation and commit to a lifetime of understanding her. She's nothing more than a child on a bio-chemistry level, so be gentle with her. Treat her like a child and listen to her. In another, deeper way, she's also wise beyond your years, and she automatically *knows* what's good for her. She *hates* to be bloated, tired and sluggish, she tells you:

That she doesn't *like* what this way of eating makes her feel like.

She doesn't *like* being weighed down with stodgy rubbish.

She *loves* clean, efficient fuel that runs her systems like a dream.

She *loves* feeling full of energy.

She *loves* feeling satisfied with her food...

A fuel that gives her an energy that she runs on all day long...no more dips! Oh no! I very clearly remember a client who said this to me "There is this wonderful feeling like my body is now running on solar energy, compared to the old, dirty fossil fuel".

Imagine that. Imagine how that feels! That's you, just a couple of weeks from now!

So now you have it...it's simple and effortless and (dare I say it?)...enjoyable! Because that is the only way to succeed at anything. Have you ever tried to be successful at something when you don't actually enjoy it? It's like walking through mud and damn near impossible. We rarely did well at the subjects we hated at school. We just don't put the right kind of positive attention there.

So see this as the **S.P.E.C.I.A.L** treat it actually is...your own little gift to your future self:

**1. SUGAR**...ditch it today!

**2. PROCESSED FOOD**...treat it the same as sugar...whether savoury or sweet, the effects in your body are exactly the same

**3. EMBRACE**...enjoying all the fats you like in your meals (it will take a while to get used to, but you will!)

**4. COMPLEX CARBS**...will be the ones that are healthiest for your body...enjoy them all...there's more than enough variety for your 5-a-day and beyond!

**5. INSURANCE POLICIES**...taking these out is vital for your success...the most important by far, is to feed yourself every day with the right food, especially in the morning, and your body will gently slip out of *CRAVE* naturally

**6. ALLOW**... yourself to make mistakes while you are learning about your body and what your triggers are...treat the next few weeks as an experiment and see how empowering that actually is to take the pressure off yourself!

**7. LISTEN**...to your body...You will hear that little *CRAVE* signal and be able to do something about it. But more than that. If you listen to her signals carefully, you will open a two-way communication that will be a steady source of comfort and nurturing that will last your whole life.

*Imagine listening and hearing a happy body. It's the best feeling in the world!*

And that really is it! All you need to do.

Do you like the sound of it? You don't have to be a meat eater to enjoy this wonderful bounteous way of eating...In fact a close friend of mine is vegan, and eats a happy low carb high fat diet (And yet not so long ago, the thought of the sugar in the cupboard was the only thing that would get her up out of bed in the mornings!).

I know this might take a while, we've got years of conditioning to unravel before you're done. But just be gentle with yourself and use this time to learn what your own triggers around food are. It may be a couple of months or so before you begin to get comfortable and familiar with this way of life, but it will happen for you!

### The Foods To Avoid...

Pasta. Bread. Rice. Pastry. All sugary foods. Most ready meals. Potatoes and most root veg including sweet potato (mainly because of the starch). Limit your pulses such as peas and beans (unless you're vegan and they are your main source of protein). Avoid all sugary fruit. Cereals and all savoury processed foods. Avoid sugary or fruity yoghurts. Or really most things that that have an advert for them! (Get savvy at reading the labels!). Avoid fizzy, sugary drinks. Beer or sugary cocktails.

## *The Foods To Enjoy...*

Once you take the processed, starchy carbs out of your body, you can start to enjoy the more complex ones such as: All the greens, (leeks, brussels, broccoli, , etc). Green beans. Red cabbage. Salad. Cauliflower. Peppers. Celeriac. Onions. Olives. Mushrooms. Beetroot (it's slightly higher in sugar at 9 g per portion, but a super-food so enjoy). Berries. All the herbs and spices you could think of. Eggs. Cheese. Cream. Meat. Fish. Nuts and seeds. Nut butters. Jacket potato skin. Pie filling. Stews. Casseroles. Pasta-less lasagne. Caulifower rice. Courgetti spaghetti. You get the picture! There's a huge variety out there for you to explore and experiment with.

You should be looking at about 50 g of complex carbs a day to be in the 'sweet spot' of feeling well fed and in *EASYBURN* at the same time. Your body will then be a Lean Mean Fat Burning Machine within the space of a couple of days.

---

*Remember the previous exercise?*

*Try it again...enjoy slowly eating a piece of cheese, or roast chicken with the skin on...whatever your favourite idea of a fatty food is, and then take a moment to really notice what your nervous system is telling you.*

*It's a deep sense of contentment and satisfaction isn't it? You could almost make a sound like a sigh it's so pleasurable.*

*And that very feeling is the ANTIDOTE to CRAVE!*

---

## *Some People Tell Me They Don't Like Fat...*

I know there may be the very rare person that truly doesn't, but for most, the truth is that they are scared to death of fat. They have been brought up from a very young age being hypnotised into believing that fat is bad.

That fat means fat.

That fat means illness and obesity and all the other major health issues we suffer from. The simple truth is that fat *storage* is bad, and now we know it doesn't happen if we are in *EASYBURN*.

If you listen to your body when you've eaten a really healthy meal, full of good fats, it will feel satisfied and fulfilled, and you will *feel* how that feels!

So you may well find you forget what the centre of the supermarket looks like. Unless you're shopping for others. You will skirt round the outside and buy everything that doesn't have an advert for it! Some people say this is an elitist way of eating and I agree...it really is! You are part of an elite club who now think in a very different way about what they eat and have taken rock solid control of their nervous system.

Who have taken themselves out of *CRAVE*. So you can now say (with a slight air of smugness),

"No thanks, I'm full."

Welcome to the club! Some say it's a more expensive way of eating, but I would really argue that it's not so.

For a start, the actual price of processed foods these days is getting more and more expensive. Especially if you consider the nutritional content you actually derive from it. Because it sets your *CRAVE* in motion, you will eat much more than your body actually needs as well. Eating a low carb high fat diet... and by 'diet' I mean *DIET* (way of eating) and not DIET!! (rubbish life!)... will diminish your appetite very quickly, so you literally won't eat anything like the amount you used to do.

The bottom line really is that veg is cheap, and always will be. The only thing I would say, is if you can possibly buy organic, then do so...there's such a wide range of organic veg now that supermarkets will provide for their customers...take advantage if you can. There is also an ever-growing number of butchers who sell free range organic meat too (you'll be hard pressed to find it in the supermarket, though...and believe me, I've tried to find it!).

So now I realise, that's all I buy these days is meat, a massive array of veg, salad, low gi fruit and dairy...and that's about it! How nice to simplify your life and your shopping list!

So what other changes can you expect to notice? When you eat like the cave girl that your body actually still is? This is by no means a comprehensive list, but some of the more usual changes that clients have told me over the last decade:

Reduced bloating.

Recovery from food obsessing.

Reduced symptoms of IBS.

Clearing of brain fog.

Having more clarity.

Better concentration.

Longer attention span.

Good night's sleep.

Feeling at peace with yourself.

Looking forward to meals again.

Feeling deeply satisfied.

Feeling freer.

Feeling euphoric.

Feeling in control.

Feeling lighter.

Less aching in joints.

Feeling happier with yourself.

Feeling proud of your new shape.

No more energy dips during the day.

Feeling more energetic generally.

Feeling more motivation to exercise.

Feeling sexier.

Losing irritability.

Feeling pleasantly surprised with yourself.

Taking up old hobbies and things you used to enjoy.

Renewed interest in cooking and feeding yourself.

Finding new 'stress solutions'.

Feeling emotionally stronger.

Easier hormonal balance.

An increased sense of pleasure in looking at yourself in the mirror.

Falling in love with your body.

Feeling stronger in other areas of life.

Easing of existing health issues.

Wondering what to think about.

There have been lots of other benefits reported to me of existing health conditions being noticeably eased. I can't comment on that. Look it up for yourself, and use your intelligence here. I wouldn't dream of going against GP or other health representative advice, but the bottom line here is that there are a wide list of issues that are caused by bad diet. Logic dictates they will be solved naturally by a good diet!

*There must be something going on here that is deeply flawed in our traditional approach to dieting, good physical health, and weight loss...*

All I know is that clients feel better in every single solitary way. Not one downside. Not one! Not a single drawback! What does that tell you? What is your body saying to you here? It will almost seem too good to be true for you.

Too easy.

Friends will comment,

"That's too much fat!"

"What are you doing to yourself?"

"That can't be right!"

"You're on another crazy diet then?"

"That way of eating is dangerous!" (Really!)

There will most likely be a mixture of jealousy, genuine concern, and maybe a little old-fashioned back biting I should think. Partners may not be that co-operative at first, and co-workers may well shove that chocolate under your nose! Oh yes they will!

They won't want you leaving the *CRAVE* club, as they know it means you will hold a mirror to their own issues with sugar and all the associated dieting issues. You have to keep the faith, which is why listening to your body's messages and trusting them is vital. *Believing* them is an absolutely essential step in the Break The Crave process.

She's *never* wrong...she *knows* what's good for her!

You will run the gauntlet of friends asking...

"Why don't you want a pudding? We *always* have a pudding...well if you're not, then I'll deprive myself too!"

Gentle, but definite...emotional blackmail. And we encounter it all the time!

It's very simple in this instance. Just tell her you're full. No need to explain about the latest thing you're doing.

Trust me.

She really doesn't care.

She's heard it all before!

There really is so much information now to back up all that I'm telling you in this little book...although not necessarily in the popular press or women's magazines (not to belittle their journalistic content one bit...but they do tend to be faddy, the latest-trend-sort-of-articles in these publications...after all fat sells!).

I mean heart surgeons, eminent professors, doctors, consultants, independent investigative journalists and geeks like me! We have done a *lot* of research between us, and I know, I absolutely know, we are right.

Look for all the recipe sites that are out there too. DITCHTHECARBS.com is a lovely site...it's comprehensive, beautiful, and has huge range of recipes. she's also passionate about the low carb high fat way of eating. (There's no affiliation by the way, I just love her site!)

Now, there's one more thing you need to know if you're a sugar girl (or guy!)....

And that is this.

> *If you eat sugar, even if it's not till you're 97, you will CRAVE it...maybe not the next day (depending on how much you ate and how sick you made yourself feel).*
>
> *But you WILL!*
>
> *And it will ALWAYS be a done deal for you.*
>
> *You are NEVER going to be a "Oh, I can just eat it in moderation" kind of a girl!*

*There Is No Moderation with addiction... Just Escalation.*

So if you *CRAVE* it. This is what you do-

Take a moment to *really notice* that feeling in your solar plexus, and give it a number. (1 being low, 10 being high) look back and see what you ate that triggered it. Or maybe where you didn't use your Insurance Policies?

There will be a reason, and you will gain a deeper insight about yourself. Sit tight and get help if necessary. Use the tapping on the website

www.breakthrough-weightloss.co.uk/tft-for-sugar-cravings

It's my absolute '*go to*' for *CRAVE* and will scramble that message from your Amygdala straight away. You'll be back off that roller coaster ride of emotions and turbulent nervous system messages soon enough.

It may take years before you and sugar wave a final goodbye. It really is everywhere.

My own personal experiences, and all the help available in

this book will give you a genuine breathing space from all of that!

You may well find you need help to get into a different mindset around your food habits. As a hypnotherapist I know only too well that therapy is the golden ticket to helping you make these powerful new changes by 'switching off' sugar craving altogether.

It also gets you in the right frame of mind to being open to trying new, colourful, exciting, interesting, pleasurable and energising foods. Find someone in your area and try it for yourself.

It's never too late to get help. I have had clients as old as 81. And as young as 12. You are never too far gone to be helped and to make changes for yourself. You have to want it. You just have to really want those changes for yourself. That is all. No striving or effort is required on your part, just an open mind and an appreciation of all the lovely food that's out there for you ☺

**For This Exercise, Find Yourself A Quiet Spot. It Will Take About 10 Minutes...**

We're going to ramp up the exercise from chapter 3 and really make that feeling work in your favour..be careful what you wish for!

**Start in the same way as the exercise at the end of chapter 3...**

**Close your eyes and imagine your favourite sugary or junk food and really notice all the sensations you experience as you bring it towards your mouth. The smell, taste and texture of it. Make it as strong as you can.**

Take a note of the feeling in your solar plexus. Give it a number from 1- 10. You may find it's quite high for you if you've really made the thought of the food as strong as you can. Don't worry, that won't last for long!

**Now...Close your eyes again, and as you imagine that particular food this time, really imagine the smell of it.**

Then see it crawling with flies. Really see those flies all over it. Hear the sound of the flies buzzing in your ears. Flies love junk and sugary food. They love to walk all over it.

**As you see and hear them. Remember where else they love to walk...on human waste. See them walking all over the filthiest toilet you can picture...see human waste all over it. SEE the human waste on those flies feet. SMELL the filthy public toilet smell coming off them.**

**NOW...See them again all over your food. Zone in to their feet and see the human waste all over their feet...ALL OVER YOUR FOOD! Now smell your food mixed in with that filthy toilet smell.**

NOW...Imagine bringing that food to your mouth, and you can SMELL it...mixed with the filthy toilet smell. Sense those flies buzzing all around your face, and they smell like the toilet. You know there is human waste from the flies' feet on that food. Put the food in your mouth now and taste the smell of it in your mouth. Force yourself to swallow it.

NOW... Open your eyes and notice the feeling in your solar plexus. Is there any *CRAVE* at all? If so...what has the number gone down to?

You can do this with every bit of junk food and sugary product you find hard to resist.

Practice this little exercise as much as you can. The power in it isn't necessarily that you will hear the flies or smell the toilet when you next encounter that food, it will just balance the books for you so that you don't feel the *CRAVE* with anything like the same intensity. That's all you actually need...it's enough to hand over the control back to you.

In that little moment when you need it.

## CHAPTER 6... MAKING THIS WORK IN YOUR LIFE

*"A girl should be 2 things: Who and what she wants"* Coco Chanel.

*Our body Simply Loves Fat. It Always Has. it Feeds Us And Nourishes Like No Other Fuel...*

As I said in the previous chapter, your body runs on it as a default fuel and always has. That's why we store it. It runs like a dream, until the fat burning system is interrupted by carbohydrates. And your body will only run on 2 types of fuel.

*Fat and Carbohydrate. Solar Energy and Fossil Fuel.*

Anything that isn't fat will be used as a source of sugar by the body, and we make insulin to metabolise that sugar. One of the main roles of insulin is to prevent your fat stores from being burned. It literally 'tells' your fat cells to stay put while it's busy using the carbohydrate fuel. So what if you're always eating carbohydrates? Your body will find it incredibly difficult to burn your fat stores. Your fat cells will do as they are told...they will stay put.

*This is why, if you eat sugary fruit, it will actually stall your weight loss*

Remember, we're not really designed to eat a lot of fruit. It's not meant to be around all that much. Unless you live in more tropical climes and then you're eating a completely different diet anyway.

> *You will feel when your body goes into*
> *EASYBURN. You'll feel your engines kicking up a*
> *gear.*
>
> *Then your energy levels will begin to rise and the*
> *fog in your brain will start to clear.*

*This Will Take Anything From 3 Days To A Week The First Time.*

It will get easier over time. The trick is to stay in *EASYBURN*, and this is where you will learn your lessons. You'll jump in and out over time though, as life happens. Celebrations, situations, holidays and off-days are always a part of life.

The main reason we 'fail' at being on a low-fat diet is that it's miserable. So if you have a way of eating instead that you really enjoy and you don't feel like you're being deprived, then you'll have much less of a reason to stay 'off plan' for long. You're loading the dice in your favour.

## I Have Noticed Something...

A few months ago I went away with my daughter, who's been eating a low carb high fat diet for a couple of years now. The food available to us at the hotel had been very limited and we'd had little choice but to eat processed carbs. On the way travelling home she said to me,

"I can't wait to get back to eating low carb"

It really struck me... You would never say *that* about a traditional Diet and Denial regime after being on holiday, now would you?!

As I said in the previous chapter, your stomach starts to shrink back down to its' natural size in just 3 short weeks. There is a very good reason for this. Processed carbohydrates expand and bloat your stomach, making the nerves that send the 'full' signal to your brain dull and unresponsive over time. They simply give up sending the message, and your brain simply gives up registering it. This is why your body can often get very confused as to whether you really *are* hungry or not.

A common complaint I hear from clients when they first come to see me is that they have a distorted sense of the true hunger message. They just have this constant craving for *something...*without really knowing fully what it is. The carbs take a lot less time to be processed by your stomach because there isn't much complexity to them. And so it's empty again in no time. It's a lose/lose situation.

Fat however... especially saturated fat... is a dense heavy substance.

It doesn't take anything like the same amount of space in your stomach that processed carbs do. It also leaves your stomach in a slow drip effect that takes hours. Its complexity means that your stomach takes a long time to process it (actually up to 8 hours!). So you will stay fuller for hours longer. Over time you will be looking for that hunger, and it just won't be there!

You will also begin a very natural-feeling process of adjusting your eating habits, as your appetite shrinks. So you'll find yourself eating your meals at a time to suit your stomach. Never starve yourself, but if you're not hungry till later in the day, then don't eat till then. It's a very modern idea to have 3 meals a day and the biggest one in the evening (a throwback to the 70's middle-class dinner party culture that we all aspired to). Before that time we would have eaten very well in the day, and had 'tea' in the evening...a sandwich, maybe...that was all.

*You'll Naturally Discover Your Appetite That Works For You And Your Body.*

Maybe you'll find that you go down to a couple of meals, or 3 small ones a day. This will take a little time. If you prefer to graze...then always have the nuts or chunks of cheese handy and honour your body's needs. The nice thing about grazing on more fatty foods is that you have a natural 'cut-off' point, a self-censorship if you will.

We literally *can't* eat too much fat when it isn't being hidden by the carbohydrates, so your palate will always let you know when you've had enough.

Personally I eat a couple of meals a day now, for the most part. I have a breakfast that looks more like your average cooked dinner. I'm on a bit of a 'stir fried greens in butter' kick at the moment...yum! And then another meal later in the afternoon. I'm just not hungry till then. That will see me through till the next morning a lot of the time. I'm not unusual either. Most of my clients report similar stories to me after the first couple of therapy sessions. They simply don't feel that hungry during the day after a hearty breakfast.

You will probably find that a snack to keep you going is all that's needed...

Think celery with sugar free peanut butter smeared on it. Or a pot of mixed tuna and mayonnaise with chopped onions etc in it. Or home-made red cabbage coleslaw that you can add grated cheese to,to your heart's content and using full fat mayonnaise? (it takes 5 minutes!). Or maybe you're a berries and clotted cream girl? So you see the picture?

This is all about playing with the rules here...throw that rulebook right out the door and all the outdated ideas of how you *should* eat. And be bold and brave...start to eat what suits you.

***"I believe that we live in a toxic food and physical inactivity environment."* Dr Kelly Brownell**

Our children will suffer the most, I fear, from this glut of over-processed slop served on our shelves and in our ever-increasing fast food eateries. They have no idea of what it used to be like, when the shops all shut at 5 o clock, and the only frozen food in the supermarket was fish fingers. And the only ready meals were freeze dried curries. We *can* teach them by example. We can show them that they can be discerning with their food choices.

If they have pizza and ready meals with their friends or eat too much of the sweet white stuff and go into *CRAVE,* you now know how to help them understand and deal with it. Information is the best thing you can give them today that will arm them against future ill health from their toxic food environment.

There are places in the world, still today, where the diet is predominantly fat and greens of various forms, and people in these cultures are healthy, strong, fit and relatively disease-free...Western illnesses are a rare occurrence, and issues like Alzheimer's and heart disease are very rare indeed. Until you get to the cities of these countries...where the western way of eating has taken its stranglehold on the population and then you see those issues starting to surface.

India is a very good example, the diet of the main percentage of the population is based on complex carbohydrates and greens of various kinds. Ghee (a kind of clarified butter) is used in almost every meal along with full fat yoghurt to flavour the food. Also nuts are eaten every day as a great source of fat and essential minerals. In the main, people are strong and healthy...this is a diet they have enjoyed for thousands of years. Unfortunately it's a different story in the cities, where childhood obesity is fast becoming completely out of control.

It doesn't take much of a leap of the imagination to know why, when (at the time of writing this book) you find out there are absolutely *no* limits on the food industry where advertising to children is concerned.

They can influence their young, soft vulnerable minds to their own un-natural ideas of what is a treat, snack or comfort food.

The kids learn from the advertisers about the food to feel cool with.

Food that all their friends eat. Food that they deserve. Food that they can eat easily because it takes no chewing. Food that will make them liked. Clever. Happy. Interesting. Included. Loved. And the kids are hooked, without the slightest clue of what's going on in their developing bodies and brains.

And they are poorly. Too heavy to run about in the playground. Out of breath running up the stairs. Unable to focus or concentrate on their school work. Teased by their classmates. When you take a moment to step outside of that insidious hypnosis of the young and impressionable, it almost appears sinister doesn't it? A report in The Times of India at the beginning of 2016 showed that there were over 15 million obese children in India, a whopping 22% of the young population! It's not much better here. The British government website (www.gov.uk/childhood obesity - updated January 2017) states "Nearly a third of all children aged between 2 - 15 are overweight or obese, and are staying obese for longer" a *third!*

> *"Human freedom involves our capacity to pause between the stimulus and response and, in that pause, to choose the one response toward which we wish to throw our weight. The capacity to create ourselves, based upon this freedom, is inseparable from consciousness or self-awareness." Rollo May*

There is one more insight I can give you that will help your understanding of you, and your body's relationship to your food...and that is the role your little *JUSTIFIER* plays.

Your *JUSTIFIER* is the last and final component to owning your *REACHING* mechanism. It might take a little time to get to know her, but she has been there all along...through your whole colourful weight loss career. And she has played a pivotal role in keeping you in a holding pattern. The Yo-Yo cycle of Diet and Denial. She is a crooning little voice, and you love to hear her.

*She's The Opposite Twin To The Little Voice You Hear In The Morning...*

*This* voice greets you as soon as you open your eyes, *she's* your *CHEERLEADER*. But she doesn't always play nice.

In fact she is strident, forceful and determined. She appears to be filled with resolve and regret all at the same time. All in the same breath, she will tell you how weak and un-motivated you are. (Boy, she can pick you apart till there's nothing left but the bones, can't she? She can make you feel lower than the floor with her vicious character assassination of your behaviour the day before... and the things you put in your mouth!).

In the very next instant she will be the strong and resolute *CHEERLEADER* who pumps you right up into believing that today we'll do better. Today we'll be full of resolve. Today we *will* stay motivated. Focused. Strong. *Determined!* She then becomes our *reasonable* voice. She can be sensible, resolute and incredibly positive.

*She will tell you that all you need to do is try harder today and you will succeed today in your weight loss wishes.*

She will tell you that it's *different* today. That you're stronger and more determined. She will make sure you completely forget all the lessons you could have learned about your body and her triggers, by denying that there was ever a problem. By assuming that the issue is just your *own* willpower.

So you resolve to listen to her reassuring, if more than a little condemning voice. She sounds like she knows what she's talking about doesn't she? You like her because she tells you that you can do this if you just get it right today.

The trouble is, your strident *CHEERLEADER* has a shelf

life. Till about 4 pm seems to be the Witching Hour...or sooner if the biscuits/cakes/fuddle/meeting snacks/ feel-good Friday/ superstar cake baker/ lunchtime grazing for interesting nibbles/missed breakfast 11 o' clock feeding frenzy don't put in an appearance first!

*This* other part of you has a very different sounding voice. Your little *JUSTIFIER.*

She is placatory. She appeals directly to your ego and has softly crooning words of encouragement in your ear.

"You've worked hard today, you deserve this"

"Just one won't matter"

"We'll just eat this then all the sugar will be gone out of the house"

"It would be rude to say no!"

"Well everyone else is so why should I deny myself"

"I'll start the diet on Monday"

"I'll go on a massive health binge in January"

"Well we've already eaten all the biscuits so we may as well forget the diet for today"

"It's my only treat/friend/pleasure in life"

"There's no harm in just a little, in moderation"

"I can't finish a meal without something sweet"

"I haven't got time to cook properly"

"I may as well eat what everyone else is eating"

"People will think I'm being picky"

"I don't like to explain about my diet to everyone"...and on and on and on she goes.

These are nothing but little stories. They are invented to make us feel better, to persuade us that we're really doing the right thing. And the thing is...we absolutely know deep down that they are not true.

Because she isn't the one that's actually causing you to cave in at the first hurdle.

*You might have guessed that your JUSTIFIER is a very clever invention by your mind to support that little tickle in your nervous system. Your CRAVE. Nothing more or less.*

She is incredibly clever with her persuasive techniques. She's had a lifetime of practice so she knows *exactly* what you need to hear. Only she doesn't actually have any *real* power over you. Not if your nervous system is quiet. Not if you take out your Insurance Policies.

Not if you take a moment when you first hear her dulcet tones during your day. It takes a little practice, but you *can* start to notice that voice...Just one small second is literally all it takes. Then you can trace that little voice straight back to your solar plexus. Right there! That's where she lives and that's where she ends.

> *Take a moment to PAUSE, jump into that sensation and own it for what it is.*
>
> *You can then start to notice something...this is exactly what is happening... Your body wants you to bridge the gap between you and whatever rubbish food is presented in front of you by making you reach out for it*

*All you have to do then? Acknowledge that.*

"Of course my body wants me to reach for that rubbish food or sickly sugary product, but I'm not going to...I'm going to choose something better for me instead!"

You will have learnt more about yourself in that little split second of *PAUSE* than you could ever imagine. You will have begun a lifelong journey of learning about yourself and the clever nervous system forces that control you. So subtle and so incredibly powerful. Understanding this intricate system of body chemical communication will literally liberate you to making a different, barely perceptible change in your thinking. This will add up, over the weeks and months, to a whole new way of dealing with your impulsive urges.

I believe that the main issue with dieting is that we don't think about our long-term weight loss goals when our Amygdala is the one in control. Remember that survival is instinctual and immediate. Long-term thinking and goal setting is another part of your brain entirely and is secondary in importance to the insistent, urgent immediacy of survival.

*Nothing* will win over it in the long run because it's designed that way. And we are at the mercy of that design. You will *never* adopt the advice from your morning-fresh *CHEERLEADER* successfully for more than a few days, or weeks at most.

You might use your super-human will-power to keep a lid on your *CRAVE* for a little while. But it takes some doing, and it will take so much out of you. It can chip away at your confidence to the point of no return. But at the end of the day it will win over you and you will end up defeated and just plain tired of it all when it does. So why fight it for a second longer?

Accept what your body needs and take out those Insurance Policies against the unbeatable *REACHING* mechanism. Arm yourself against your little *JUSTIFIER*. You know what will happen then?

Those two voices will simply fade like mist into the past, and you will very quickly forget that you ever used to have this long running script. This schizophrenic three way conversation with the Ghosts of Persuasion in your head. There will just be you. Satisfied and fulfilled. And did I say empowered? I think I probably did. So now you are.

You have everything you need to successfully lose weight not just for now, but for your lifetime.

You can re-visit this book and all the help that's in it as much as you need to. Treat the next 6 weeks as the experiment and you will be truly amazed at what you learn about yourself.

After all, your diet is the most fundamental relationship you have with your body. It is deeply intimate and personal, and you will have your very own triggers that set you off in a flash. If you *learn* from them, rather than treat them as a failure you will have the best Insurance Policy of all...*self-insight!*

You will really get to know your little *JUSTIFIER* as you become more aware of your triggers, addictions and your own quirky food relationship. Once you really *own* your habits you will become well and truly armed and dangerous!

So then...you can arm yourself against yourself. Simple as that!

**Now You Know How: You PAUSE. In That Little CRAVE Driven REACHING Moment.**

You take just one split second to take a step back. To sit on your own shoulder and to notice in *clear and perfect* detail exactly what is going on with *you.* Exactly how clever your *JUSTIFIER* can be...to really *hear* her voice and what she's saying to you. To *feel* what that craving sensation is actually like in your solar plexus.

But today, in that split second *PAUSE,* you can decide to make a different decision. To simply walk away. Just for that moment. Just for now. Simple and easy. No negotiation. No anxiety. Just a calm and easy understanding of yourself and your own little moment in front of the shelves in the supermarket, the workplace or the kitchen.

> *If you follow the S.P.E.C.I.A.L Break The crave System and use your Insurance Policies you simply can't go wrong. You will lose weight...without any striving or sacrifice whatsoever.*

I know at first it may take a leap of faith. That commitment to taking out the 6 week experiment and trusting the Break the Crave System and just going for it. What lies on the other side of those 6 weeks is sheer relief, you'll see.

Oh and you'll be about a dress size down by the way too. Did I mention that?

So you'd better have something in the wardrobe ready and waiting for you to triumphantly jump into. So you can parade around your bedroom doing the Happy Dance!

*Catching Yourself In The Mirror At Every Opportunity With A little Secret Smile On Your Face.*

Begin to break those rules and be an inspiration to those around you. Remember that others will *always* eat in a way that's right for them. You can just eat in a way that's right for you. Right?

If you're worried about breaking those so-called rules around the 'dangers' of fat, or how set meal times should be. Or what weight loss should *be* like...take a quick look around you, just to give yourself a gentle reminder of what's *not* working. Traditional dieting is *not* working.

> *If I had a pound for every time a client told me about a friend who had been successful at losing weight at a slimming club I'd be a very rich woman. Because the story always ends the same...they have put it all back on again!...Where's the success in that?!*

It's pure failure and back to the drawing board. Back to a painfully slow and, let's face it, boring process to lose weight again. Yet again.

*I wonder what we would all be doing with our free thinking time as successful women in the west, if we weren't constantly obsessing about our latest calorific intake??!*

And what about all that self confidence that wouldn't have been slowly eroded away over the years by diet failures that were seen to be caused by a lack of inner strength, or motivation on our part?

What if we were brought up inhabiting strong, confident bodies, and had nothing but respect for them? If we were taught that our bodies were beautiful and we could eat all the lovely fats they wanted without any fear or guilt?

As a mother of a daughter now in her late 20's, I was really aware that I didn't want her to inherit this poisonous, pernicious self-loathing. This obsessive diet mentality that swathe so many of us in a cloud of illusory promises of thin-ness if we just *tried harder!* Followed by the inevitable self-sabotage that simply obscures who we really are and what we are really capable of being and achieving. We are at an unprecedented time in our history where we have more rights, freedoms, education and autonomy.

*And Yet we Waste Years Of Our Lives Thinking About a Phantom Menace Called fat That Doesn't Even Exist!*

I'm pretty sure in generations to come that they will look back at our time with incredulity. Shaking their heads in disbelief over what we did to ourselves and our bodies. How we held ourselves down with a straight jacket, heavy as concrete, formed from self-loathing and chronic body consciousness.

Let's break the rules from today, and show our daughters especially (but son's too, of course, I know they have their own issues ..I'm just writing from a woman's perspective as we feel the pain of body shaming disproportionately so). That they can inherit bodies that are strong, resilient, lean and disease-free. Give them the freedom to simply think about something more interesting instead.

And it's not too late for us either! Once we free ourselves from the debilitating shame of living in a body that doesn't feel like ours. Once we feel the freedom to be ourselves. Once we recognise that if we can do this...we can do *anything* we set our minds to!

And once we finally, once and for all, tell the food and diet industries where to shove it and begin to choose our *own* way of eating. *Then* we will finally be free to take the next step. On the other side of the Break The Crave System is a life lived fulfilled and satisfied, liberated and owned completely by you. What *will* you do with it? The rest of the story is up to you!

It's only your food...and yet that is *everything!* It's where the story of your whole life begins and ends! No more and no less.

As a very last little P.S to this book, I want to help you with what I know to be the last tiny piece of the jigsaw puzzle, and that's getting into the right mindset. And I mean *really* getting into the right mindset!

Because you might just need a bit of a hand to make that *PAUSE* moment work for you. To give you a gentle but powerful nudge in the right direction towards a calm and simple sea change in how you feel about those foods you want to eliminate out of your life, and your body once and for all.

So this is what I would like to give to you...it's a very powerful download that has the *PAUSE* moment built into it.

It's Deep Dive Relaxation (as hypnotherapy is also often called) and I would like to gift it to you for free.

Then you'll have everything you need to successfully, happily, easily, effortlessly... in fact, *joyously*...lose weight for now and into the future.

Use this link to the download...it will be available for as long as you need it, as often as you do...enjoy!

https://soundcloud.com/breakthrough-weightloss/weightloss-hypno-download

## *Here's To A Lifetime Of Eating In A Bubble Of Pleasure...Every Single Day!*

Now...you can go and find something more interesting to do with your time because if you can do this...you can do *anything* you set your mind to, can't you?

*These Are The Last 2 Exercises In The Book, And They Are By Far The Most Powerful...*

they are clever little tricks that you can use in other areas of your life too if you wished. For the purpose of this book, I've helped you to take control of your eating urges, but you're just as able to take control in other situations in your life too. Your little *JUSTIFIER* is present whenever you buy a dress that you probably shouldn't do, or a pair of shoes you know you'll never wear! There are a thousand other situations too, so...

---

**DAY 1 ... Notice all the times in your day that your little *JUSTIFIER* comes into your mind. What words does she use with you? What's the tone of her voice like? Write down as much as you can. You might find that it's difficult to keep up with her, and that she's actually there a lot more often that you realise!**

Don't try and change anything, or even argue with her. Just observe what happens for you. Sit with her and just notice her. Treat her like a little friend that's come to join you for a moment.

---

**DAY 2 ... Do the same thing, but with your *CHEERLEADER*. She is a different voice from your *JUSTIFIER*, so just take a note of the times when you recognise her voice, when she speaks and the words she says. Again write it down, and don't do anything to change her. Just invite her in.**

Take at least a week to do this first exercise so you to get to build a really good picture of your day-to-day thinking around food.

**Alternate listening to these little voices in your day. Take your time if you're enjoying the exercise. Notice what happens as you get to know them more intimately.**

You might even be able to recognise who's voice they are? Or maybe where they are located..behind your ears or on your shoulder perhaps?

**The key is to be gentle with yourself here. There's no time limit to learning about these two!**

For the second exercise, begin to bring the *PAUSE* into the moment when your little *JUSTIFIER* is making her presence known.

**IT ONLY TAKES A SECOND TO *PAUSE*...**

You might find it helps to actually say the word "*PAUSE*" quietly to yourself. Notice the feeling associated with her voice in your solar plexus. Don't do anything with it. Just notice all these subtle little influences going on for you at that particular little moment. How does that make you feel? What would you like to do with it? Sit on the moment for as long as you want. You're in control now...you can do whatever you like with that little moment. The choice is entirely yours.

The more you practice the *PAUSE* mechanism. The more you will be able to sit on your own shoulder and recognise those little twin voices for exactly what they are. The more in control of your eating habits you will become...

**Can you feel that? Can you see the immense power that you hold in that little moment in time?**

**When you're just able to say:**

**"No thanks, I'm alright for now"**

*Some Of My Favourite Low Carb Life-Savers!...*

Cutting the carbohydrates out your diet doesn't have to be a major life- overhaul for you.

In fact, you'll have a much better chance of successfully changing over to a new way of eating if you can adapt the dishes you already enjoy now. You're much less likely to feel like you're missing out that way, and you can still eat with the family without much fuss. They might even get curious to try out this new way of eating- especially once they begin to see you looking so healthy and full of energy!

There are some great replacements for the carbohydrates on your plate nowadays. These are the most common ones:

1.  **CAULIFLOWER RICE- Steam cauliflower florets in the microwave for a couple of minutes.** Then use a potato masher to break them up into smaller pieces. Mix them with butter and put them into a crispy jacket potato skin, covered with melted cheese. You could also use them as a rice replacement with that kind of texture or grate them into a pan of boiling water and cook for a couple of minutes if you want a more authentic rice-like texture...you really won't be able to tell the difference.

2. **BRAISED LEEKS- Split them down the centre and peel the outer layers open.** They make perfect pasta sheets for a lasagne. I saw this done for the first time by the Hairy Bikers, and their guests were completely unaware they weren't eating the real thing!

3. **CELERIAC- Is a real unsung hero in my book!** Its' texture is similar to swede, so will need a little more cooking than most root veg. However it's very low in starch and carbs, so is great for making chips, or roasting in oil and salt. Blend it with butter for the perfect celeriac mash. It's actually a member of the fennel family, which isn't normally a taste I'm very fond of, but I love it. I highly recommend that you give it a try! (Use it as a filling in jacket potato skins too as an alternative to cauliflower florets for a really authentic texture).

4. **COURGETTE- Last of the carb replacement giants-** Put this humble little green through a spiraliser to create 'courgetti spaghetti'. You can pick up a decent spiraliser for a few pounds...mine cost just £6 from the local supermarket. All you need do is push the courgette through the spiraliser blades to make ribbons of 'spaghetti' that cook in a couple of minutes for the perfect accompaniment to bolognaise, carbonara and tomato sauces. How cool is that?!

*I've Also Added A Couple Of The Most Useful Recipes For You...*

They are super-simple and you can adapt them to suit your needs in lots of ways:

**First Up Is:**

*The Incredibly Simple PIZZA DOUGH:*

**Ingredients-**

85 g mozzarella cheese

2 tbsp cream cheese (full fat)

120 g almond flour

1 egg

pinch of salt to taste

Shred the mozzarella cheese, add it to the cream cheese and almond flour and mix together. Microwave on full power for 1 minute. Fold in the egg and salt (you can use your own flavourings to taste). Microwave again for another 30 seconds. I recommend using greaseproof paper to line a baking sheet as the dough can be a bit sticky. Then either roll it or simply flatten the dough out with the palm of your hand. Cook on 220c for 12 minutes. Turn half way through for a crispier texture on both sides. I would recommend playing with the amounts of flour and cheese slightly to suite your taste.

You can then add your favourite toppings to suit and put back in the oven for 5 minutes or so...as long as it takes to cook the cheese! I spread a layer of cream cheese on the dough rather than tomato paste and then add chopped olives, mushrooms or sliced pepperoni, and grated cheddar as a topping. The nice thing is that I can take it to work and graze on it cold during the day...it's deliciously filling but with none of the stodginess of traditional pizza.

*Making a thinner dough will give you crackers, or a thick dough will give you more of a bread consistency*

### Spread Low Carb 'Nutella' As A Topping If You Want Something Sweeter...

**Ingredients:**

1 tsp sweetener (Splenda works well for me, but you might prefer one of the others...avoid aspartame though!)

1 small tsp 70% cocoa powder

2-3 tbsp pouring cream.

Mix all the ingredients together in a small bowl. This will make a soft creamy texture to spread on your pizza dough crackers! You could also create a chocolate sauce topping by adding a little more cream to it. My pudding on Christmas day was meringue made with sweetener rather than sugar, topped with chopped strawberries and chocolate sauce. Heaven!!

*The pizza dough was first created by Libby at DITCHTHECARBS.COM and is called Fat Head Pizza*

You could always post your own version of these recipes in the facebook support group **My Diet-Less Life.**

I'd love to see you there and hear what you thought of this book!

Much love

Bridgette x

# ABOUT THE AUTHOR

Bridgette qualified as a complementary therapist in December 1997. She also qualified in nutrition and diet and anatomy and physiology. She has been a full-time therapist for the last 20 years. She has a special interest in how the nervous system affects our behaviour, and how we can control it for better physical and mental health.

She has worked with a wide range of clients over the years both privately and in the corporate world, as well as in drug and alcohol services, mental health charities, women's' and youth aid organisations and a wide variety of public sector organisations. She runs workshops all over the country teaching people how to gain control over their nervous system responses, using a wide range of tools to create emotional resilience and mental well-being.

She studied and qualified in hypnotherapy in 2006, and now works as a full-time hypnotherapist at her clinic, The Park Hypnotherapy Centre, on the outskirts of Nottingham city centre.

She blogs as often as she can, and speaks to a variety of groups on the subjects of health, weight loss and nutrition; she also talks extensively on the subject of hypnotherapy and its' benefits in mental and emotional well-being.

# OTHER AUTHORS WITH GREEN CAT BOOKS

**Lisa J Rivers –**
Why I Have So Many Cats
Winding Down
Searching (Coming 2018)

**Luna Felis –**
Life Well Lived

**Gabriel Eziorobo –**
Words Of My Mouth
The Brain Behind Freelance Writing

**Mike Herring –**
Nature Boy

**Glyn Roberts & David Smith**
Prince Porrig and the Calamitous Carbuncle

**Peach Berry –**
A Bag Of Souls

# OTHER AUTHORS WITH GREEN CAT BOOKS

**Michelle DuVal** –
The Coach

**Elijah Barns** –
The Witch and Jet Splinters – Part 1: A Bustle In The Hedgerow

**David Rollins** –
Haiku From The Asylum

**Sean P Gaughan** –
And God For His Own

**Brian N Sigauke** –
The Power Of Collectivity

**DO YOU HAVE A MANUSCRIPT READY TO BE PUBLISHED?:**

**SEND A SAMPLE OF YOUR WORK TO**
**books@green-cat.co**

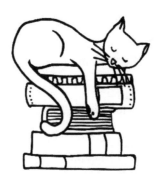

GREEN CAT BOOKS

**www.green-cat.co/books**

CPSIA information can be obtained
at www.ICGtesting.com
Printed in the USA
LVHW05s1547290518
578844LV00037B/1052/P